Live Better flower essences

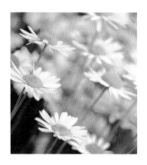

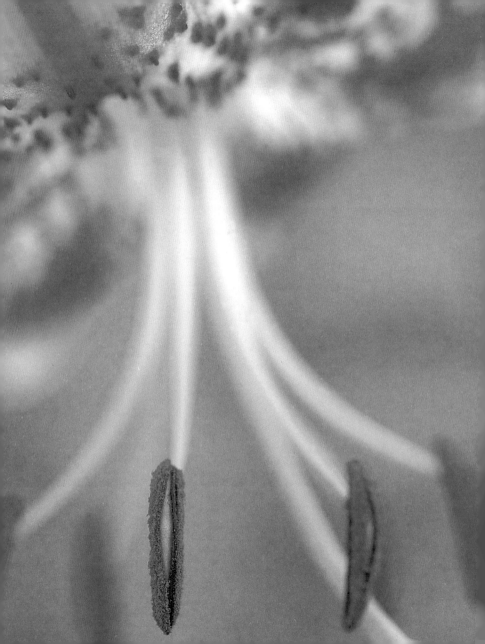

Live Better flower essences

remedies and inspirations for well-being

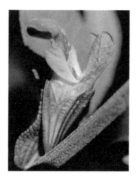

Clare G. Harvey

DUNCAN BAIRD PUBLISHERS

LONDON

Live Better: Flower Essences
Clare G. Harvey

"Flowers speak of love silently in a language known only to the heart", is a truth that my grandmother taught me. This book is dedicated to my grandmother and my mother Eliana, with gratitude for the wisdom they generously shared with me.

First published in the United Kingdom
and Ireland in 2006 by
Duncan Baird Publishers Ltd
Sixth Floor
Castle House
75–76 Wells Street
London W1T 3QH

Conceived, created and designed by
Duncan Baird Publishers Ltd
Copyright © Duncan Baird Publishers 2006
Text copyright © Clare G. Harvey 2006
Commissioned photography copyright © Duncan Baird
Publishers 2006
For copyright of agency photographs see p.128, which is to
be regarded as an extension of this copyright.

Managing Designer: Manisha Patel
Designer: Justin Ford
Managing Editor: Grace Cheetham
Editor: Ingrid Court-Jones
Picture Research: Susannah Stone

British Library Cataloguing-in-Publication Data:
A CIP record for this book is available from the
British Library.

ISBN: 978-1-84483-293-4

10 9 8 7 6 5 4 3 2

Typeset in Filosofia and Son Kern
Colour reproduction by Scanhouse, Malaysia
Printed by Imago, Malaysia

Publisher's note

Before following any advice or practice suggested
in this book, it is recommended that you consult
your doctor as to its suitability, especially if you
suffer from any health problems, special conditions
or you are pregnant. The publishers, author and
photographers cannot accept any responsibility
for any injuries or damage incurred as a result of
using any of the essences or remedies described
or mentioned herein.

contents

Introduction

Flowers have always been a source of pleasure and happiness, and can play an important role in promoting harmony in mind, body and spirit. Instinctively you already know and have experienced the therapeutic power of flowers. How many of us have found solace strolling among fields or in gardens filled with flowering plants? We feel uplifted by the sight and aroma of fresh flowers, and often give them to someone who is unwell, or as a gesture of celebration or commiseration.

Our existence is becoming increasingly artificial. It is easy to feel isolated from the natural environment when we live and work in towns and cities. We are also exposed to more and more stress, which has been recognized as a major source of ill-health and unhappiness. Stress tends to be infectious. If you work in an environment full of anxious, frazzled people, it is difficult to keep calm. Add on family and financial pressures, and stress can overload your system. But orthodox medicine offers little relief for stress-induced problems.

It is in this climate that many of us are now taking responsibility for our own health and well-being by seeking new ways in which to manage stress creatively. Increasingly, people are turning back to nature and to old tried-and-tested remedies.

Flower essences have existed since prehistoric times. However, it was Dr Edward Bach, a Harley Street physician, who last century reminded us that the essences of flowers and plants were available to help us heal ourselves. Since his pioneering work, there has been a great resurgence of interest in flower remedies, and producers have started making essences from an extraordinarily diverse variety of flora from all over the world, including England, North America, Asia, the Amazon jungle and the Australian outback.

It is a great pleasure to be able to introduce you to the wonderful world of flower remedies. In the following pages you will find essences to address many of life's challenges, and with their support, I hope you will be able to manage your life more effectively. It is very rewarding to see how flowers can come to the rescue!

Chapter One

flower essence wisdom

Flowers are nature's way of decorating the earth in a wonderful expression of colour, shape and the most exquisite fragrances possible. It's as if the designer of our planet has taken delight in painting the world alive with vibrant hues that range from one end of the colour spectrum to the other.

Since ancient times humankind has responded to flowers with awe, instinctively appreciating their magical and sacred qualities, and marveling at their variety. Our ancestors chose flowers as a medium through which to express their innermost feelings and elevated thoughts. Flowers feature in many stories, myths and legends of gods and goddesses –

even the creation of the world has been attributed to some of our most spectacular floral species.

Natural wild flowers used to be abundant in fields and woodlands, and they still are in some areas, such as jungles, rainforests and mountain valleys. Each flower has its own, individual essence that has a specific purpose. Some are said to heal and others, such as the rose, promote love and romance. The orchid enhances our connection with the spiritual world, while the lotus is an aid to reaching enlightenment. It's as if Mother Nature has presented us with these invaluable gifts not only to gladden our hearts and lift our spirits, but also to heal our being.

WHAT ARE FLOWER ESSENCES?

Ancient peoples, who lived closer to the natural world than we do today, had a direct relationship with their environment. They not only found physical nourishment in the flowers and plants that grew around them, but also discovered that these had properties which could promote emotional and spiritual healing. When our ancestors sipped the dew from the petals of flowers that had been warmed by the first rays of the morning sun, they noticed that it had an incredible, uplifting effect on their spirits, calming their minds and cooling their emotions. Curious to know more, they investigated further and discovered that a different effect was obtained from each of the amazing variety of blossoms available.

They learned through observation that the highest concentration of a plant's life force was in its blooms at the peak of its growth. Maybe they also sensed that there was a form of energetic imprint beyond a flower's colour, shape and scent, which was only usually visible to birds and insects. Each flower had its own unique signature to attract certain insects or birds to pollinate it and ensure its continued survival.

Some medicine men and women of the time who were gifted with the ability to "see" this invisible energetic pattern devised a process of capturing the flowers' energy so that they could use it to help to heal their tribespeople. They floated blossoms in spring water outside in the midday sun, which acted as a catalyst to draw out the flowers' life force and healing qualities. This potentizing process allowed a flower's etheric imprint to be transferred into the water. The imprinted water became known as the "mother essence", and was preserved in alcohol to be used when needed. This mixture is known as the flower essence or remedy.

Flower essences are significantly different from other natural remedies. While essential oils, homeopathic medicines and herbal tinctures use a physical part of a flower or a plant, essences contain only the energetic patterning or imprint of the flower – its positive, life-giving energy.

HEALING ENERGY AND THE SUBTLE ANATOMY

The concept that all life is made up of a complex web of integrated and interchangeable energy, and that through this interwoven web we are all interlinked, was widely accepted by the ancients.

Most civilizations had a healthy respect for the force of nature, which was called *qi* by the Chinese and *prana* by the yogis in India, both of whom had a clear understanding of this energy. The cultural records of the Hawaiians, too, reveal that they were acutely aware of the powerful and magnetic life force that permeated their islands. They referred to this healing energy as *mana* (spiritual power), and believed that it was omnipresent in the natural world and that it particularly heightened the energetic qualities of flowers.

To understand how flower essences work, it's important to learn first about our subtle anatomy – which contains the blueprint for our perfect health – and how a flower's healing energy interacts with our own.

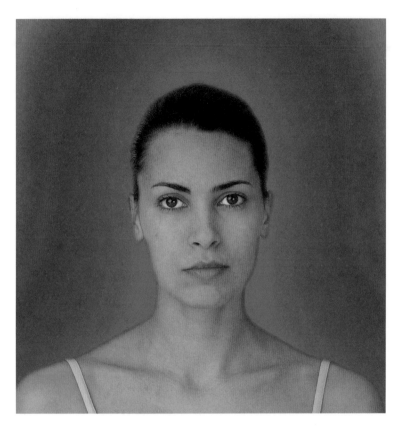

This person's aura is hazy, having come into contact with the energy fields of more than 100 people at a natural health show.

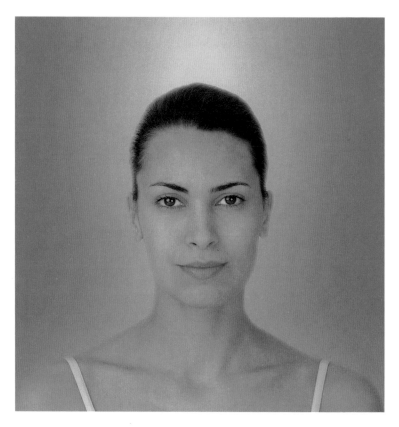

The same person's aura after they have taken a flower essence –
clearer, revitalized and much brighter in colour.

Many healing traditions acknowledge that every thing living possesses a subtle energy field. In us, the more smoothly this energy flows, the better the function of the whole being. Modern science has at last caught up with this ancient knowledge, as research in theoretical physics has shown that every form of matter emits dynamic energy, which has a unique vibrational pattern and frequency.

When disturbance occurs in this patterning, disharmony and "dis-ease" result. This reverberates at cellular level because the fundamental particle itself is a pattern of pure energy, which in turn has an effect on our physical, emotional, mental and spiritual energy levels.

Energy-collection centres in the body called chakras are like a second nervous system, acting as transforming stations to regulate the body's internal energy flow. They also regulate the aura, which is a luminous energy field surrounding and emanating from inside the body as a result of its biomolecular activity. This is preceived by some as a halo of light. The colours and density of a person's aura reflect their vitality and state of health.

HOW FLOWER ESSENCES WORK ON AN ENERGETIC LEVEL

As we have already mentioned, we are made up of a complex structure of interchangeable energy, which is linked to the cosmos and runs through the body via the subtle anatomy, and it is this which holds our blueprint for perfect health. It is therefore clear that when our energy is blocked, stressed or disturbed, we need to turn to the natural world for answers, for this is the moment when vibrational reprogramming is needed at cellular level to re-establish harmony in our blueprint.

As humankind has a profound relationship and a natural resonance with plants and flowers, it is not surprising that they can affect us in a positive way.

The ability of flowers to heal is thought to reside in their special vibrational qualities. Each flower transmits its own unique energy pattern or essence. When the appropriate essence is used, this acts as a catalyst to return our energy back to its original state of harmony by restoring its natural frequency. There is a flower or a combination of flowers to match any of the numerous imbalances that the human organism may experience. In this way flower essences work to re-align and shift the subtle anatomy back into its former state of balance and allow the body's self-healing process to activate.

When you consult a flower remedy practitioner, they will ascertain the compatible resonance by dowsing or intuitive diagnoses. They will then be able to accurately pinpoint the correct essence or combination of essences for you. Acting in its own specific way, the essence is attracted to the area in most need of attention, flooding it with positive energetic information. The area soaks up the healing energy like a sponge. This process is known as "sympathetic resonance".

Not only do flower remedies have particular resonance with chakras and the aura, but they also directly affect the physical body. As toxicity in the form of disharmonious frequencies such as negative thoughts, emotions and patterns of trauma are transmuted and flushed out of the system, the body can regain its healthy blueprint.

Life engenders life. Energy creates energy. It is by
spending oneself that one becomes rich.

SARAH BERNHARDT

(1844-1923)

Energy is eternal delight.

WILLIAM BLAKE

(1757-1827)

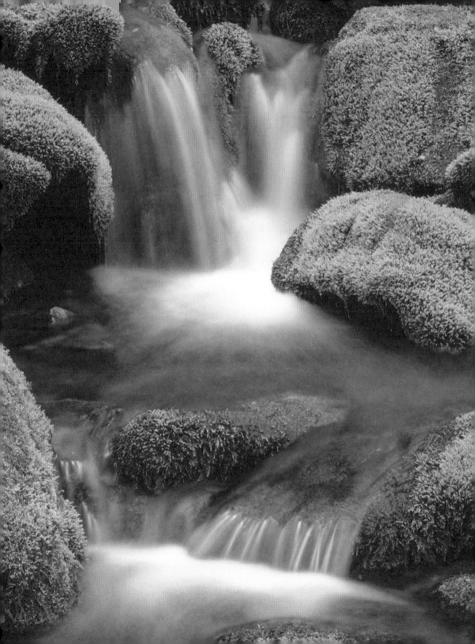

HISTORY: ANCIENT KNOWLEDGE

The ancient Egyptians harnessed the healing power of flowers by blending flower essences to treat a wide variety of illnesses. They also perfected the art of distilling flowers to obtain the oils which today we call aromatherapy oils, by collecting sun-drenched dew from flower petals to use in combination with essential oils.

They believed that ill health was not just a physical matter, but the result of an imbalance in the mind, body and spirit. Ancient records show that they created a complex system of medicine that skillfully combined flower essences with other healing modalities to treat ill health holistically.

In Egyptian society exotic, ornamental and healing gardens were created to delight the gods, and some flowers were regarded as sacred. Blue and white lotuses were offered at festivals for the gods in the hope that the deities would protect and grant a long reign to the pharaoh. The iris was a symbol of royal power, its three petals denoting wisdom, faith and valour.

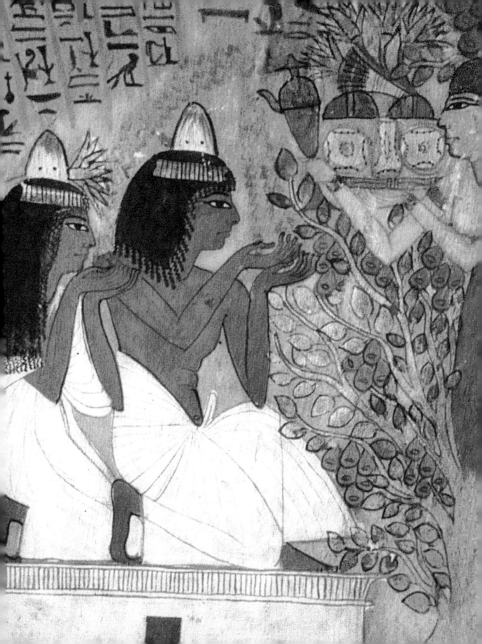

HISTORY: A COMPLETE SYSTEM OF MEDICINE

It is thought that the Egyptians rediscovered the lost art of flower essences. Their high priests — "the knowers of the secret arts" — realized that the spirit of a plant was encapsulated in its flower essence and could be used for healing. Early Chinese, Indonesian, Mesopotamian and African civilizations recognized and utilized flower essences to treat emotional states. The Minoans of Crete, a highly cultivated and spiritually developed people, floated chosen flowers in water during sacred ceremonies and sipped the water to cleanse themselves of negative thoughts and feelings. They also placed flowers in bowls of water around the sacred space to protect and enhance the ceremony.

High up in the Himalayas where the "valley of the flowers" is traditionally resplendent with exotic flowers, the natural medicine system of Ayurveda evolved. Over 5,000 years old, Ayurveda acknowledges the therapeutic value of flowers. The lotus takes place of honour in

Ayurvedic healing ceremonies, in which petals are floated in water that is then drunk or anointed on the body.

In the Americas, according to an ancient Peruvian legend, flowers possessed their own healing song, and the Seminole Indians tell of a shaman who heard and learnt a flower's healing song while wandering in the woods, and took it out into the world.

Over time, the knowledge of flower essences was largely lost again, but it was preserved by secret brotherhoods, such as the Essenes in Sinai, until it was rediscovered in the fifteenth century (see p.26).

Aboriginal Healing Art

The Australian Aborigines, considering themselves to be direct descendants of the original inhabitants of the earth, also kept safe the knowledge of the healing power of flowers. They believed that their ancestors had sung the world alive, calling the flowers and trees into being with sacred words that wrapped the planet in a web of song. The web had to be recreated constantly by the elders walking along the songlines to keep creation alive.

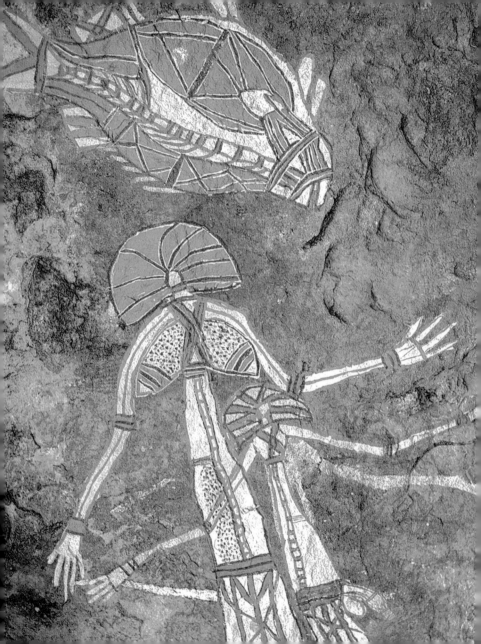

The Aborigines are custodians of a spectacular range of wild flowers that bloom throughout the year. In the tribal mythology of the Nyoongah of South Western Australia, flowers embody the colours of the "rainbow snake", the creator spirit who allowed the Sun woman to breathe warmth into the ice-covered world. So flowers reminded them of how precious life was, as flowers are displayed in all the colours of the rainbow.

The Nyoongah peoples ate whole flowers that were drenched in dew, gaining the healing qualities of the flowers' essences as well as their nutritional benefits. If the flowers weren't edible the people absorbed their healing vibrations by sitting quietly among them.

The medicine man or *mobarn* of the tribe held ceremonial healing rites to resolve specific emotional and physical imbalances. He would prepare an earth pit containing hot coals layered with flowers sprinkled with water, and place a kangaroo skin on top to create a sauna effect. After an all-night ritual in the pit, the person emerged at dawn "reborn," the sickness having been replaced with the spirit of the flowers.

HOW FLOWER ESSENCES HAVE DEVELOPED

The power of flower essences was rediscovered by the Swiss doctor and author Paracelsus (1493–1541), who collected the morning dew from blossoms to treat his clients' emotional imbalances.

In the 1920s, an English physician, Dr Edward Bach, became dissatisfied with medicine and searched for a simple system to treat the root-cause of illness, which he observed to be mostly shock and stress. He found his answer in flowers and blossoming trees. Using himself as a guinea pig by allowing negative states of mind and emotion to overtake him, he was drawn intuitively to the flower whose essence made him experience the opposite emotion. He built up a repertoire of 38 essences that are widely used to treat individual responses to stressful events according to each patient's personality type.

In the last 25 years, there has been a revival of flower remedies from all over the world, including the Australian bush, the Himalayas and the Amazon jungle.

Ian White, a fifth-generation herbalist, explored the powerful flowers used by the Aborigines, and brought out Australian Bush Essences, a range that includes Emergency Essence, and Electro Essence – a notable combination to counteract the negative effect of cellphones, computers and electromagnetic pollution.

Richard Katz of the Flower Essence Society in the USA conducted intensive research into the use of flower remedies as antidotes. He has brought out a cream that has extraordinary healing capacities.

Judy Griffin of the Petite Fleur Texan range has focused on flowers that strengthen the immune and nervous systems, and clear the negative effects of stress.

Lila Devi of the Master's range encourages becoming master of your own life. She has concentrated on blossoming fruit and vegetables, which are especially effective for mothers and children.

Andreas Korte, the German pioneer, found his own ecological method of encapsulating the flowers' energy in water and discovered some unique orchids in the Amazon jungle.

WHAT FLOWER ESSENCES CAN DO FOR YOU

The extra stresses and strains of contemporary life have demanded new ways of handling the problems we increasingly face. Many highly sensitive people, who are able to tune in to the vibrations of plants and flowers. have responded by investigating the healing qualities of additional flowers, especially those traditionally regarded to have sacred healing powers. This has resulted in a veritable explosion in the use of flower essences and they are now being offered extensively as a profound healing modality.

The most significant factor about flower remedies is that they are an extraordinary gift to enable self actualization. User-friendly and multifaceted in approach, they have the ability to completely turn life around in a gentle yet powerful way.

Flower essences clear deep-seated shock and stress, often penetrating to the root of ill health so that our innate self-healing mechanism can re-establish itself.

Not only do they clear ingrained habit patterns, but they are also preventative and educational – the more sensitive and in touch with ourselves we become through using flower essences, the quicker we are able to correct and prevent negative patterns from forming before they develop into something more serious or deep-rooted.

Through continuously releasing the blockages that interfere with and hold back fulfillment of our true potential, flower essences empower us to be better able to respond to and benefit from the challenges that modern life presents.

Practical by nature, some flower remedies work not only emotionally, mentally and spiritually, but also physically on problems we experience as a result of the weakening of the immune and endocrine systems, such as allergies, hayfever, skin complaints, hormonal imbalances and electromagnetic pollution.

In their wisdom, ancient medicine men and women handed down to us a precious and invaluable tool to use on our journey through life in this uncertain world.

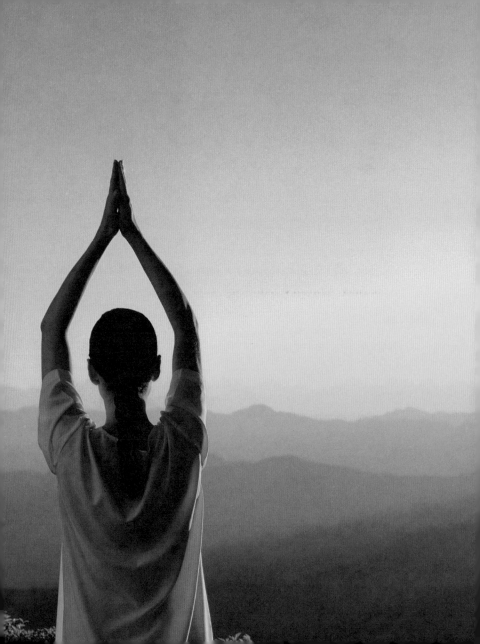

Harmony in eating and resting, in sleeping and waking:
perfection in all you do. This is the path to peace.

BHAGAVAD GITA

(1st–2nd century bc)

Chapter Two

prescribing flower essences for yourself

Flower essences are self-adjusting — more is not necessarily better, except in an emergency situation. They work on the homeopathic principle that less is more — a slow, continuous reminder of how the body *should* be is highly effective.

After reading the flower essence repertoire (see pp.44–125), you will be instinctively drawn to particular essences. Choose the one that resonates most with your situation.

Flower remedies clear grief, relationship problems and emotional upheavals, and help you to handle stress more effectively. When you are making significant career and life-style changes, or you face a transitional stage of life, such as becoming a parent, simply taking an essence to lift your mood will create an immediate shift in energy and vitality. However, to treat deep-seated trauma or ongoing chronic issues, it is best to consult an expert in the field.

Flower essences can really help in acute situations, so it is advisable to keep a remedy such as Australian Bush Emergency Essence, or Pear Blossom (which is especially potent for children) to hand for emergencies. In such cases, you can take it often: between once every five minutes and once an hour.

TAKING ESSENCES

There are many ways to take flower essences. You can ingest them, or use them externally in creams or oils for the skin, or add drops to your bath. You can also absorb them by spraying them into the air or onto your aura.

The traditional way to take essences is as drops under the tongue or mixed with a little water and sipped. The standard dosage is seven drops to be taken morning and evening, and more often in emergencies and situations that are extremely stressful.

To avoid consuming alcohol or when treating babies and children, you can gently rub the essence onto the skin on the pulse points, on the inner sides of the wrists, the forehead or the soles of the feet. This is equally effective as ingesting them.

You can also create a remedy bath by adding a few drops of the required flower essences to your warm bath – this is akin to being totally steeped in liquid energy. Relax and soak for at least 30 minutes, by which time you will have readily absorbed the energy of the essences.

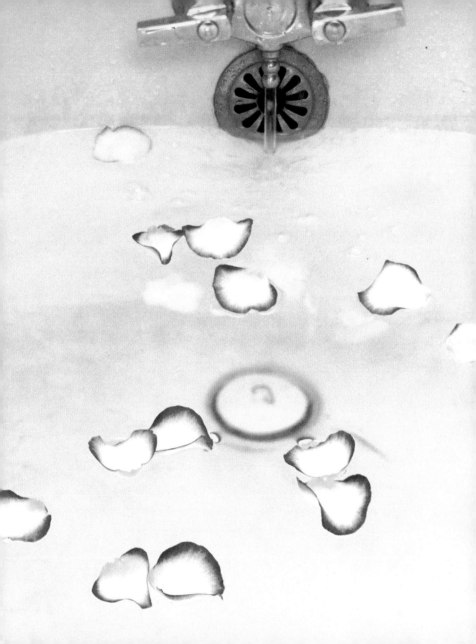

FLOWER ESSENCE COMBINATIONS

Combining essences is a fine art – the more the maker is in tune with the flowers, the more effective and potent the combination will be. Targeted at specific common problems, they are a good introduction to flower essences. Many producers offer combinations of single essences, which are designed especially to help us to meet the challenges of day-to-day life. The combinations come ready to use in dosage bottles. The suggested way to take them is to have two to seven drops in the morning and evening as often as required.

Some popular combinations are:

Dynamis Essence Combats exhaustion, burnout and loss of drive; brings energy, enthusiasm and stamina.

Cognis Essence Increases clarity, focus and concentration; especially useful when studying and taking exams.

Stop Smoking Blend Clears emotional dependency and the addictive patterns associated with smoking.

Reduce Stress Blend Gives great support for handling the build-up of daily stress.

Travel Essence Aids travel by combatting jet lag and time disorientation.

Woman Essence A combination that is used successfully in Swiss and Brazilian hospitals to treat hormonal imbalances, and problems with menstruation, pregnancy and the menopause.

Allergy/Intolerance Blend Combats reactions to foods, chemicals, pollens and grasses.

Combinations for the Bath

Add seven drops of your chosen combination to the bath, along with a few drops of your favourite essential oils for a wonderful treat.

Emergency Essence A recommended pick-me-up that refreshes and revitalizes after a long, tiring day.

Calm and Clear Essence or **Hibiscus Essence** Is beneficial before retiring at night as it relaxes the system sufficiently to encourage deep and harmonizing sleep.

Electro Essence Is good for clearing the build-up of electro-magnetic pollution that we absorb while working on computers.

SPRITZES

When flower essences are used in spritzes that are sprayed into the air, they clear the build-up of stale, stagnant energy and improve the atmosphere of a room. In sprays, flower remedies are combined with aromatic essential oils to provide a boost to your energy and sweeten the air. By spritzing into the auric field and subtle anatomy, you can diffuse the negative effects of an emotionally charged environment.

Some suggested sprays are:

Space Clearing Spray Clears the immediate environment. Add some Electro Essence to dissipate radiation and electromagnetic energy at work, especially when using your computer and your cellphone.

Harmony and Balance Spray is a feng shui spray that reduces stress and anxiety, harnessing beneficial energy to recharge stagnant energy.

Spirit Lift Spray This is an exotic combination specifically for women, which refreshes and uplifts the spirit and enhances sensuality.

TAILOR-MADE COMBINATIONS, SPRITZES AND CREAMS

Working with flower remedies is fun. Make your own combinations by mixing single essences together, or add them to spritzes. Decide which issues you would like to address, then choose the essences to which you are most drawn (see repertoire, pp.46–119). Use no more than seven essences in any one blend to start with.

Combinations

Fill a 30ml/1fl oz dropper bottle with 10ml/2 tsp brandy, then add 3–4 drops of each of the chosen essences and fill up with spring water. This is your dosage bottle from which you take seven drops morning and evening.

Here are a few combination recipes to try:

Re-balance Combo Mix equal amounts of Almond Blossom, Apple Blossom, Green Rose, Old Blush and Wild Rose to rebalance energy and maintain its balance.

Meditation Remedy Blend equal amounts of Lotus and Paradise Lily to still your mind.

Happiness Remedy Blend equal amounts of Cherry Blossom, Wild Violet, Magnolia, Orange Blossom and Nootka Rose to enhance your inner smile.

Feminine Enhancer Mix equal amounts of Orchid Queen, Cherokee Rose, Tibetan Rock Rose, Bird of Paradise, Lehua and Frangipani to balance femininity.

Spritzes

Tailor-making your own spritzes means you can personalize the remedies to your requirements. In a 50ml/1¾fl oz spray bottle put 4–5 drops of each essence, plus a few drops of your favourite essential oils and 15ml/1 tbsp vodka, shake vigorously to disperse the oil and then spray around your own energy field and surroundings.

Uplifting Mist to energize and lift your mood: Sun Orchid, Cherry Blossom and Nooka Rose essences mixed with a few drops of may chang and orange oil.

Protection Spritz is an energy shield to protect your aura. Blend Angel of Protection Orchid, Sage, Aloe Vera and Self-heal essences, mixed with a few drops of juniper or geranium oil.

Creams

Although flower essences are generally taken orally, they are very effective blended with essential oils in a botanical cream or aloe vera gel base for local application, either as a face cream or for medicinal purposes.

The flowers are selected for their therapeutic properties, which are absorbed through the pores of the skin into the bloodstream, and delivered to the area where they are most needed.

Some lovely combinations are:

Bird of Paradise Beauty Cream An exotic, de-stressing, anti-ageing and deeply moisturizing cream with Bird of Paradise and Orchid essences to encourage a woman's confidence in expressing her inner beauty and sensuality positively.

Floral Relief Gel and Floral Arthritis Gel Quick-acting, cooling aloe vera gel combined with essences made from a variety of Himalayan flowers to give relief from backache, headaches, painful periods, sprains, injury and itchy eczema. The arthritis gel cools the swelling and discomfort of painful joints.

The human body is vapour, materialized by sunshine
and mixed with the life of the stars.

PARACELSUS

(1493–1541)

Chapter Three

repertoire of flower essences

The flowers in this repertoire have been chosen from among the thousands of fabulous flowers that can be found on the planet today. There is no doubt that all flowers are unique and awe-inspiring, but some hold extra significance for us, as they did for our ancestors who also appreciated the sacredness and understood the special healing qualities of flowers. These blooms have become part of our heritage and we can now benefit fully from the revival of their use as a healing art.

In the following pages you will find stories, myths and legends concerning an array of flowers hailing from many diverse areas and cultural traditions. From the exotic orchid that grows in the Amazon jungle to the humble daisy found in the English countryside, they all reveal their energetic qualities and demonstrate how useful they can be in supporting our lives today.

Many flower-essence makers have produced interesting and informative booklets, which describe in great detail the special healing attributes of each of their remedies. These booklets offer a deeper understanding of what is now available and enable people to make appropriate and informed choices about flower essences for themselves.

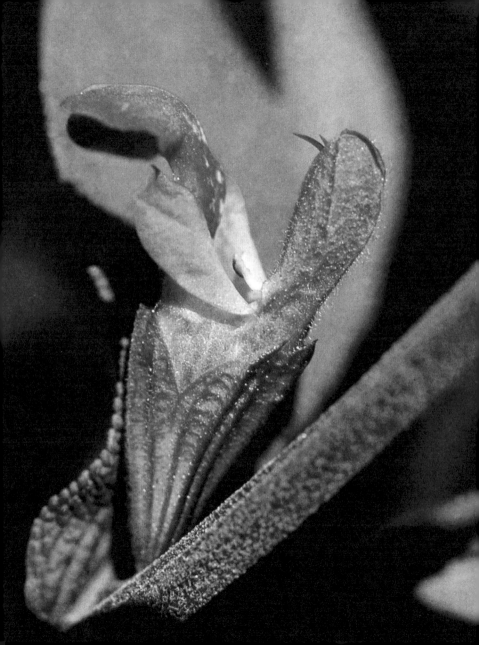

SAGE: CLEANSING AND PURIFYING

The sage family (*Artemesia*) is named after Artemis, the Greek goddess of hunting and the moon. It was one of the most highly valued medicinal plants, and hunters of old rubbed sage into their skin to cover their scent.

Native North Americans knew of the power of sage and burned it believing its sweet smoke would carry messages to the spirit world. The plant is still ceremonially burned in smudging rituals to banish negative forces and cleanse participants of toxic thoughts and emotions, thus clearing the way for connection with Spirit. Sage leaves are included in medicine bundles and pouches, and are also used to cover the floor of the circular, domed structure of the Sweat Lodge, where purification ceremonies take place. The Lakota people wear garlands of sage around their ankles, wrists and necks as protection while taking part in the sacred rites of passage known as the Sun Dance.

Sage Essence Cleanses and purifies energy, restoring our inner rhythm and balance.

ALOE VERA: REVITALIZATION

According to legend, this succulent plant with its wonderful healing properties grew in the Garden of Eden. Its upright, flame-shaped flowers were known as "wands of heaven" by the Native North Americans. Originating in eastern and southern Africa, aloe vera was used by the ancient Egyptians, and is depicted in their art. Cleopatra bathed in its juice to preserve her delicate skin.

Aloe vera has been used both internally as a strong purgative, and externally as a superb healer of bruises and scars. It is well known for its cooling and anti-inflammatory effects. Today the plant grows in tropical climates around the world.

Aloe Vera Essence Restores inner balance, replenishing and nourishing internal energy and renewing vibrancy. Recommended for workaholics and those who burn the candle at both ends, and for people who have a tendency to neglect their physical and emotional needs, and suffer from exhaustion and burnout.

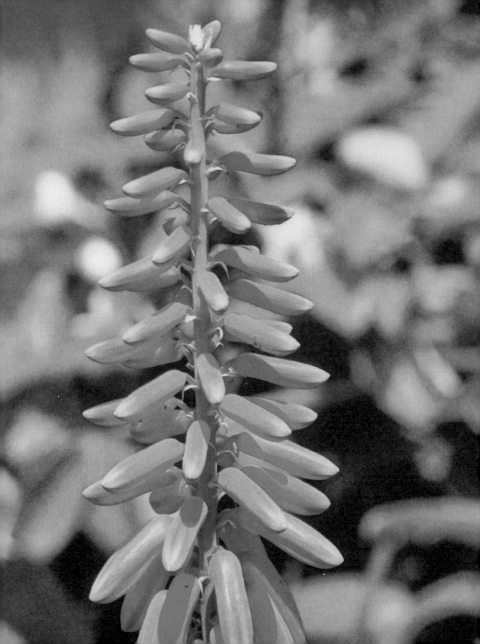

HIBISCUS: COMPATIBILITY AND CALM

The beautiful, large flowers of the hibiscus come in a range of shades from pink to red to yellow, and are characterized by their long stamens.

Originally from China, the red hibiscus is the national flower of Malaysia. In Indonesia the flowers are found in offerings that decorate ceremonial objects. On the island of Bali, men traditionally wear red Pucuk hibiscus flowers behind their ears on romantic engagements. Hawaiian men use the red Kokio hibiscus to announce their marital status — a flower behind the right ear means they are happily married; a hibiscus behind the left ear that they are single, and a flower behind each ear indicates that they are married but looking for someone new. The rare, endangered, yellow *ma'o hau hele* hibiscus is the state flower of Hawaii.

Hibiscus Essence Works on calming women's nerves and inner core, supporting the *qi* of the nervous system.

Red Hibiscus Essence Enhances intimate relationships by evoking warmth and responsiveness.

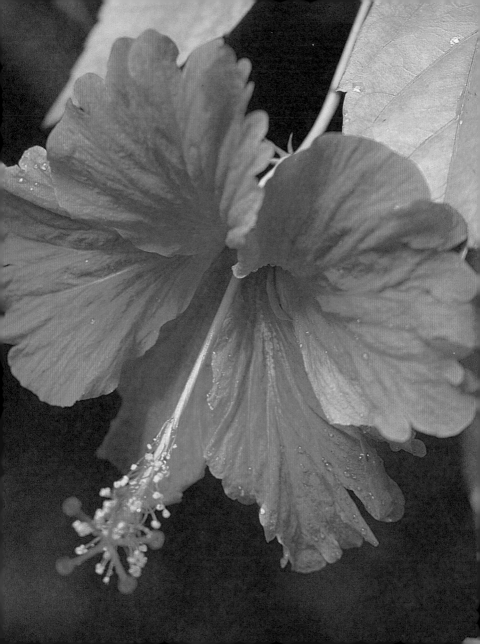

STURT DESERT PEA: GRIEF AND PROFOUND HEALING

Sturt desert pea is the floral emblem of South Australia and one of the country's most stunning native plants — it has brilliant red flowers with glossy black centres. An extraordinary feature of this plant is that it needs to be subjected to the harshest of environmental changes, such as a bush fire, to trigger germination, and this can take up to 40 years.

Revered by the Aborigines and known as the "flowers of blood" the red blooms symbolize the blood of their ancestors who perished in the struggle to survive. A sad legend tells of the "birth" of this plant and hints at its healing qualities.

A young warrior Wimbaco Bolo fell deeply in love with Purleemile, the beautiful bride-to-be of a cowardly old man named Tirtha. Wanting to be together, the young couple eloped and joined Wimbaco's father's hunting tribe across the lake. When Tirtha requested Purleemile's return, he was invited to do battle with

Wimbaco to win her back. Refusing, Tirtha decided to bide his time. In the meantime Purleemile had a handsome baby boy, who was the tribe's pride and joy.

One day, Purleemile received songs of foreboding from the spirits. Alarmed, she pleaded with Wimbaco to flee the area, but her proud husband wouldn't listen. One night, Tirtha and his men came and took delight in killing the whole tribe, including Purleemile and her baby.

When Tirtha and his men returned a year later to gloat, they found the lake was dry and full of salt. Terrified, the men fled leaving Tirtha behind, but instead of the bones of Wimbaco's tribe he found a carpet of vibrant red flowers. While he stood transfixed by these flowers, a loud voice suddenly denounced him for spilling the innocent blood of Purleemile, Wimbaco and their little boy. "Their blood will live forever," the voice boomed, and then a spear came down from the sky and impaled him to the spot. It is said that the salt lakes are the dried tears of the song spirits and that the Sturt desert pea will flower for ever on the salt plains.

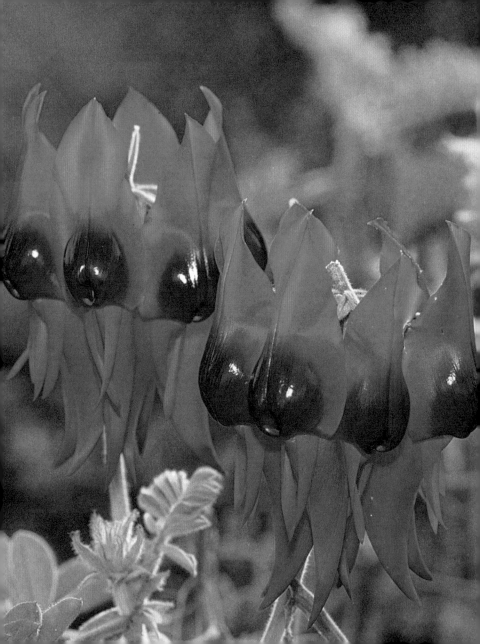

Sturt Desert Pea Essence is a deep-acting, powerful remedy, which can be profound in initiating major life changes. The long life of Sturt desert pea seeds gives an indication of the flower's ability to clear and heal stored pain that has not previously been released. It heals old emotional wounds and dissolves deep-seated sadness that has been held in the system for a long time.

The main area that is affected by the presence of deep sorrow is usually the lungs, where grief can cause breathing problems such as bronchitis and asthma. Sturt desert pea is recommended for when we are unable to let go of the emotional pain and anguish of separation, whether in divorce or the loss of a loved one, or at the end of an affair, or even in cases of first love. Expressing emotion is something that Western men find particularly difficult because of cultural conditioning.

The action of Sturt desert pea is multifaceted, helping to fight viruses, and bacterial and parasitic conditions, as well as clear emotional trauma. It is a good general tonic for the physical body, and it supports finding practical solutions to life's problems.

WARATAH: COURAGE AND STRENGTH

The origins of this exceptionally stunning and sacred flower can be traced back 60 million years to Antarctica, but today it is found only in Australia. The Aborigines call it waratah, which means "most beautiful", and Australia is known as the "land of waratahs." The flower has often been depicted in Aboriginal art. The Tharawal tribespeople drink its nectar not only for pleasure but also for its curative powers and the strengthening effects it has on the tribal elders and young children.

It is said that when the Aborigines first saw the early white settlers, the king of the Burragorang tribe generously presented the governor with a waratah flower – their most sacred bloom – as a peace offering. To the Aborigines the waratah embodied the qualities of survival and tenacity that they, as Australian bush dwellers, had in abundance. They saw how difficult it was for the white people to adjust to the harsh climate and reality of their new home, so they also gave them the waratah flower to help them to adapt more easily. Totally taken with this flower, the early white settlers thought it was the most magnificent plant they had ever seen and called it the glory of the Australian bush.

The waratah is so very important and significant in Aboriginal culture that their folklore has some wonderful legends about its "birth".

Long ago a beautiful Aboriginal woman, who wore a coat ornate with the red crests of the gang gang cockatoo, was deeply in love with a young warrior of her tribe. All was well until a neighbouring tribe trespassed on their land and her lover went into battle.

She spent seven days on the sandstone cliff waiting for him to return. When he failed to come back, her tears formed rivulets in the sandstone from which bush fuchsia and boronia flowers sprang up. She was unable to live without him and her spirit passed through a crack in the sandstone. From there grew the most beautiful and perfect of all plants. Its serrated and pointed leaves were said to represent the lover's spear, while the glowing red flower symbolized the woman's red coat. Thus the lovers were joined together in spirit in one splendid flower.

Waratah Essence This is a powerful healing essence of great importance. It is a quick-acting, emergency remedy for those going through the dark night of the soul, bringing courage and tenacity to anyone feeling suicidal or suffering from despair or deep depression.

Waratah helps people to discover and call upon deep reserves of inner faith and strength that they already possess. It encourages them to adapt, and enhances their ability to cope with crises and to tap into previously learned survival skills, revealing their own hitherto undiscovered inner resources.

Essence of waratah has been used very successfully in Brazilian hospitals, where it is used by cardiologists treating heart imbalances, ventricular failure and mitral valve insufficiency. It has also helped to arrest the development of glaucoma, and in some cases has reversed it. Waratah can also be used to fight chronic depression where a black cloud descends on someone without warning, leaving them unable to lift out of it.

In the language of flowers waratah suggests prosperity, and the essence promotes positivity and abundance.

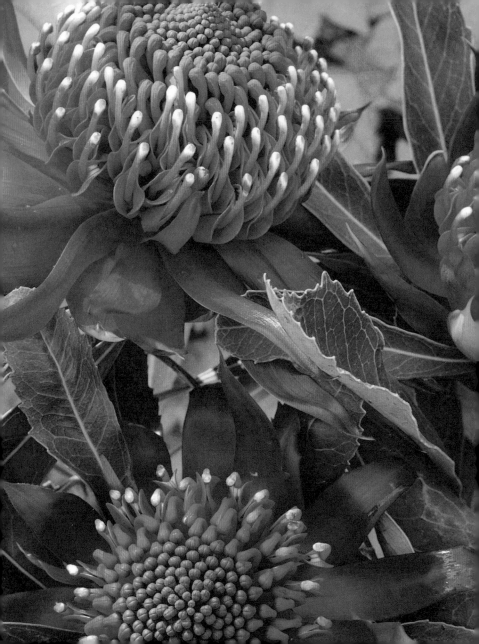

SELF-HEAL: HEALTH AND VITALITY

Self-heal flowers range in colour from soft, light pink to radiant magenta, and their nectar is second to none in the opinion of discerning bees.

The Druids picked self-heal when the star Sirius was rising and placed it on their altars for healing purposes. Medieval herbalists called it the "heal-all" of plants because of its universal healing properties. Early American settlers called it "Heart of the Earth", and for centuries it has been used for skin problems and has been taken as a regenerative tonic. The famous herbalist Nicholas Culpeper (1616–54) praised self-heal as a "special herb for inward and outward wounds."

Self-heal Essence Encourages a healthy sense of self, awakening vital inner forces. Aids multi-level healing on physical, emotional and spiritual levels, producing a deep sense of well-being.

Self-heal Cream Is beneficial as a soothing, nourishing and rejuvenative moisturizer. It is anti-inflammatory and deeply regenerative for all skin conditions.

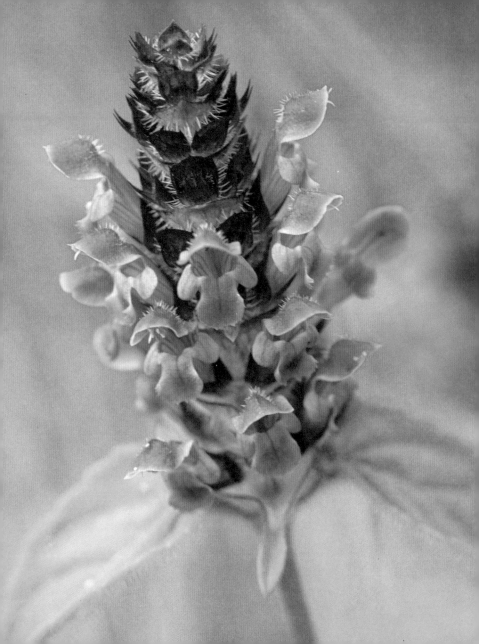

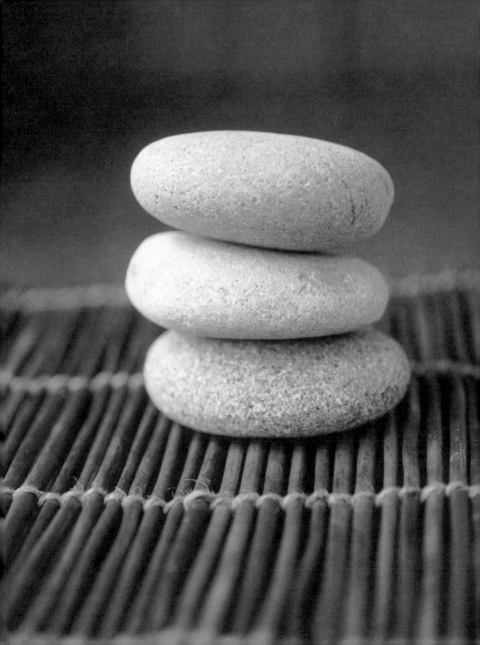

So divinely is the world organized that every
one of us, in our place and time, is in balance
with everything else.

JOHANN WOLFGANG VON GOETHE

(1749-1832)

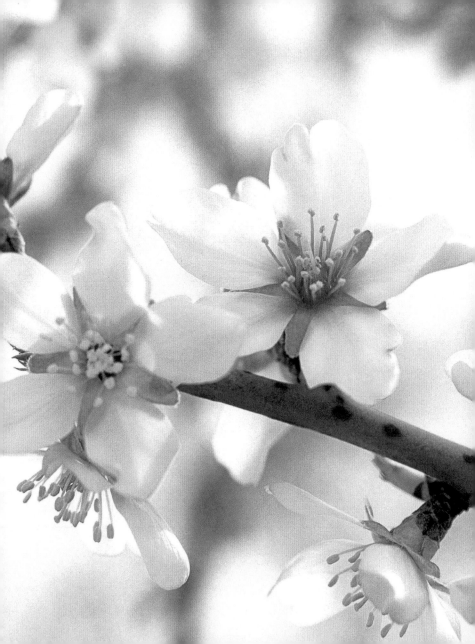

ALMOND: RE-BALANCE

The almond tree is native to central Asia, although some almonds were found in Tutankhamun's tomb in Egypt. Ancient Egyptian women ate sweet almonds to gain weight, and when Arabs made long journeys across deserts they sustained themselves with almonds, dates and water.

A Greek story tells of a time when true love transcended death. When a maiden was abandoned by her lover, she was heartbroken and died. Out of pity the gods changed her into an almond tree. Her lover then returned and was devastated. Grieving, he embraced the tree and it burst into flower.

In the language of flowers, almond blossom signifies hope eternal.

Almond Blossom Essence Helps us to find the middle way when we are exhausted and overwhelmed. Calms the mind and the nerves, harmonizing the mind, body and spirit. Also beneficial for pre-teenage children, as it stabilizes mood swings and restores emotional balance.

MAGNOLIA: SELF-APPRECIATION

Descended from a very ancient species of plant, magnolias have been discovered in fossil deposits dating from 5 million years ago. The American magnolia has huge white flowers and a heavenly lemon scent. It is a floral emblem of both Louisiana and Mississippi. The magnolia is known as the "secretly smiling flower" in Russia.

In China the cultivated magnolia symbolizes the gentleness and feminity of a beautiful woman, while the wild variety represents perseverance and dignity.

Magnolia Essence Is designed for those who have little self-belief and feel undeserving. On a nutritional level this can lead to a lack of absorption and assimilation of food. Magnolia encourages a positive and a healthy self-appreciative attitude, especially of the finer qualities of the personality. It also helps integration.

Japanese Magnolia Essence Blends masculine and feminine energies within, clearing women of vulnerability and over-dependence on men, and balancing the feminine energy within men.

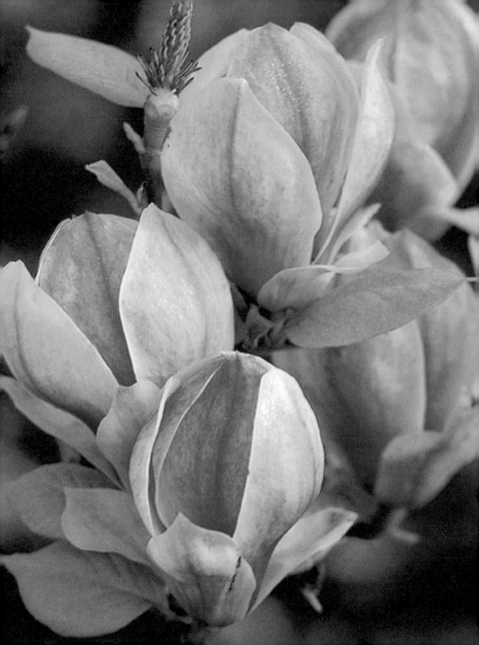

BIRD OF PARADISE: INNER BEAUTY

Perhaps one of the strangest and most flamboyant flowers native to Africa, this brilliant blossom was likened to an exotic bird of paradise in flight when its brightly coloured plumage and fan-like tail is seen flashing through the treetops. The jungle shamans say the bird floats in heaven and feeds on dew. The flower slowly unfurls its fabulous bright orange and dark blue petals one by one, a sight that sunbirds and sugar birds cannot resist. They pollinate it by transferring the pollen gathered on their breast feathers as they move from flower to flower. The blossom is also known as the crested-crane flower as it resembles the bird of that name.

In the language of flowers the bird of paradise represents freedom and magnificence.

Bird of Paradise Essence Helps us to see our true self and discover our "inner beauty" regardless of our outward appearance. It teaches us self-acceptance and to follow our inner vision unerringly.

Bird of Paradise Cream See Creams, p.41.

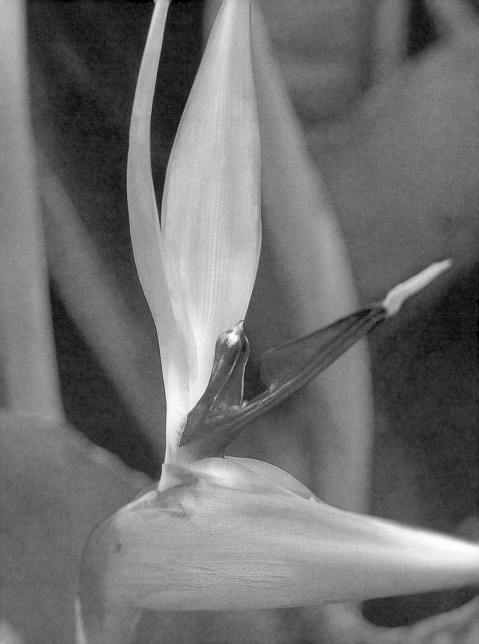

IRIS: INSPIRATION

The iris is known as the "eye of heaven", and grows in more colours than any other flower, which is why it is associated with the Greek goddess of the rainbow, the messenger of the gods who splits light with her speed. According to fairy folklore iris fairies manifest themselves in the colours of the rainbow, stimulating inspiration and psychic purity.

In the Minoan palace of Knossos, irises were painted around a relief of the priest-king as a representation of his deity. In Egypt, too, the iris was an ancient symbol of royalty and majesty. It was also highly valued for its perfume and used as an offering to the gods. The perfume industry in Florence, Italy continued to use the iris well into the eighteenth century.

Iris Essence This is a fundamental remedy for restoring and revitalizing the inner life of the soul and harmonizing it with nature. It aids the soul's mission to build a rainbow bridge between spirit and matter so that we can become truly alive and vibrant.

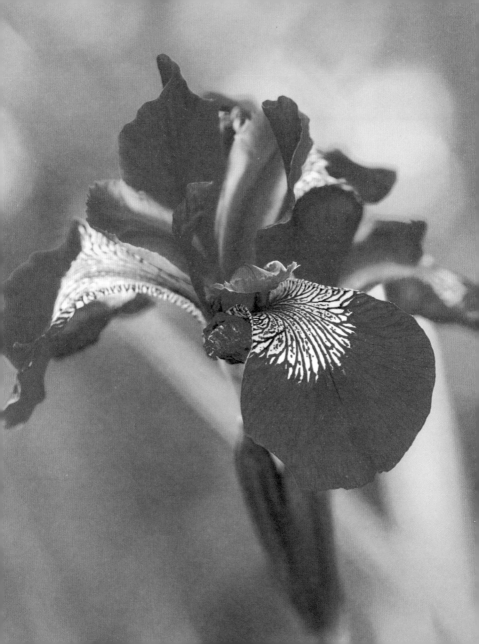

DAISY: CLARITY

A favourite flower of wood nymphs, the daisy resembles an eye, and it was used by primitive medicine men and women to treat visual problems.

The Assyrians used the daisy not only to heal the eyes, but also in a tincture which, when added to oil, was said to turn grey hair back to its original colour. Depictions of daisy-like flowers have been discovered on the heads of some golden hair pins that were found in the Minoan palace of Knossos. The daisy has also been painted on Egyptian ceramics. In Anglo-Saxon times daisy potion was added to holy water and potentized with incantations.

There is an old English saying that spring has not arrived until you have set foot on twelve daisies, and to this day, a favourite childhood pastime is to make daisy chains or garlands on warm summer days.

Daisy Essence Helps us to collect, clarify and synthesize our thoughts so that we can gain an overview. It is ideal for both adults and children who are learning new skills.

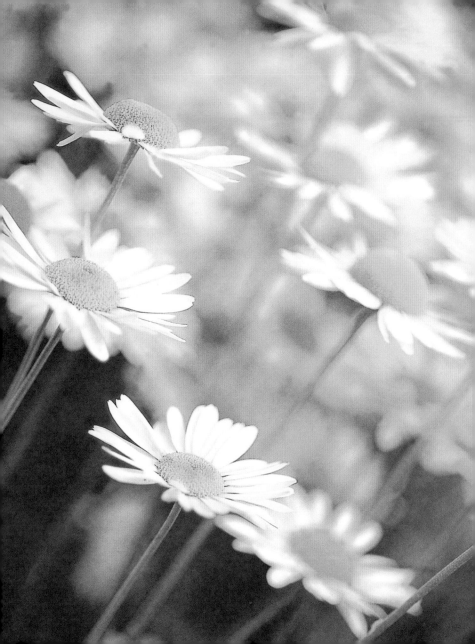

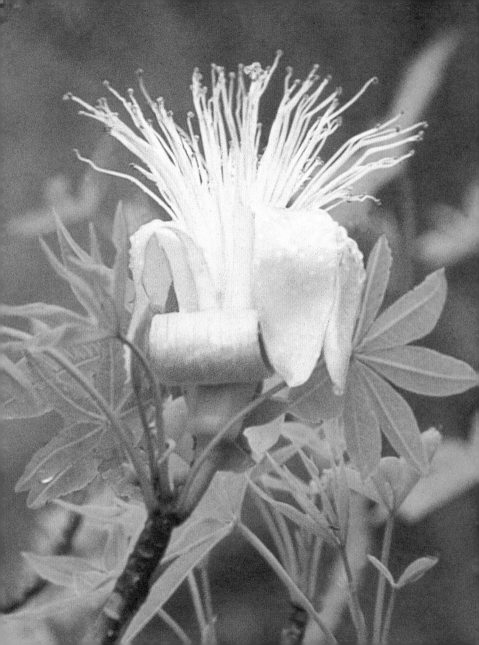

BOAB TREE: INNER FREEDOM

The ancient boab tree, found only in the north-western region of Western Australia, has large, creamy white flowers with long stamens that exude an aroma similar to the tuber rose, The younger boab trees often grow in a circle around the mother tree, which they are eventually engulfed by and merge with — an indication of the flower's potency for clearing enmeshed family patterns.

This healing quality was utilized by Aborigines in their traditional birthing practices. A tribe would collect boab flowers for a woman giving birth during the flowering season. The mother-to-be would find a quiet spot in the bush and dig a shallow pit, lining it with the blossom before giving birth. The first contact the child had with life was being surrounded by fragrant boab flowers with their powerful healing ability to clear the negativity passed down from previous generations.

Boab Essence Effective for treating genetic illnesses originating in learnt emotional patterns passed down through the family, giving freedom from the past.

CHERRY: CHEERFULNESS

Wild cherry blossom is a vision to behold in the spring, a sight that the Japanese, with their deep love for this flower, have honoured since ancient times. Their most sacred places, the mountains, abound with cherry blossom and are associated with Ko-No-Hana, the goddess of spring and abundance, and daughter of the mountain god Oho-Yama. When her spirit takes possession of the cherry tree it allows her to descend from heaven to earth bringing purity, simplicity, hope and new beginnings.

At the spring flower festival of Hanami, the Japanese hold flower-viewing parties under the blossoming trees in the temples and shrines, to celebrate the cherry's vitality. Prayers are offered to the flower goddess to ensure a plentiful harvest.

Cherry Blossom Essence Promotes cheerfulness and light-heartedness, clearing moodiness and feelings of being emotionally out of control. In children, cherry replaces sadness with happiness and heals the trauma caused by the separation and divorce of their parents.

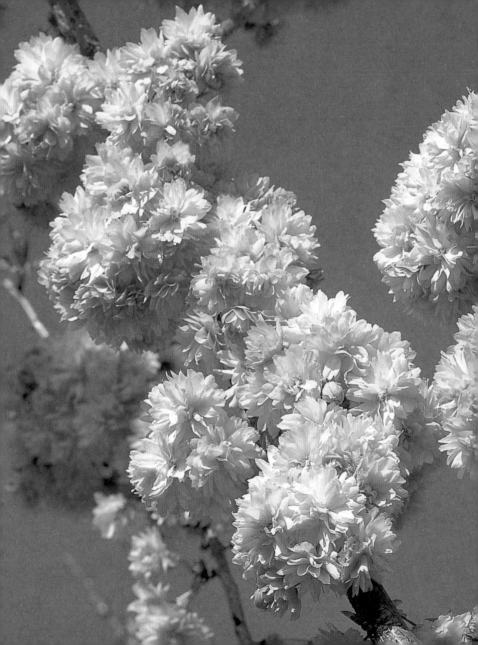

Happiness is a butterfly, which when pursued, is always just beyond your grasp, but which, if you sit down quietly, may alight upon you.

NATHANIEL HAWTHORNE

(1804-1864)

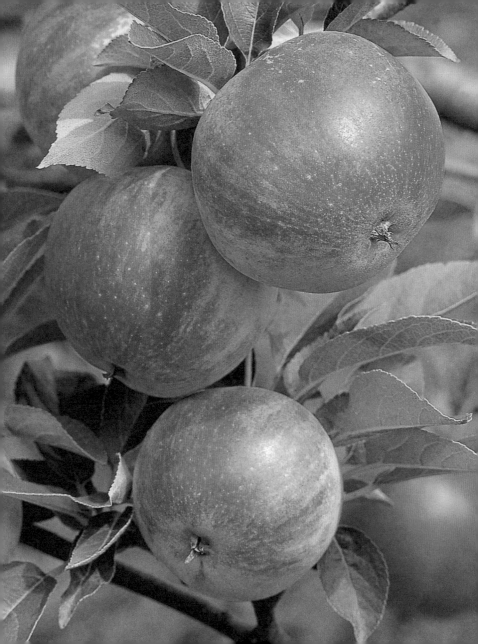

VIOLET: OPTIMISM AND TRUST

Native to ancient woodland, violets form a vibrant carpet of purples and blues in springtime. The rare fen violet is perhaps the most beautiful variety, its bluish-white flowers suffused with a mother-of-pearl sheen.

Violets have been used to make perfume since the times of classical Greece. A Greek legend tells of Io, a wood nymph, who was loved by Zeus. To protect her from his jealous wife he changed her into a sacred cow, but she wept when he gave her only coarse grass to eat. When Zeus saw this he changed her tears into sweet-smelling violets that she alone was allowed to eat.

In medieval Britain violets were used to treat insomnia and depression. Since then, the flowers have been made into garlands, nosegays and posies as a symbol of faithfulness and taking a chance on happiness.

Wild Violet Essence Brings a sense of optimism, and encourages us to explore new options while keeping a balance between cautious and courageous decision-making. Enhances trust in the face of the unknown.

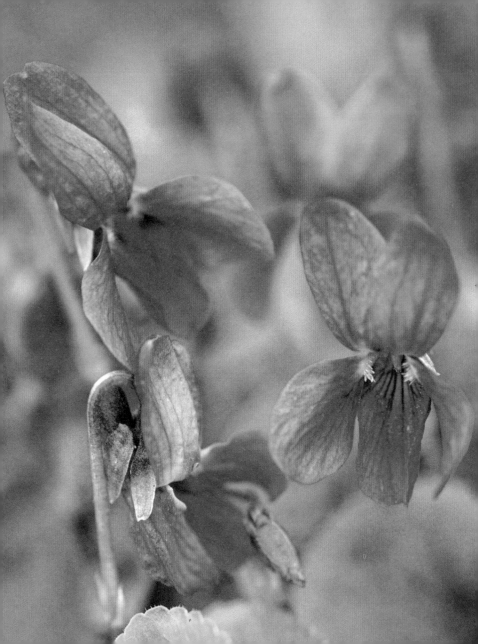

ORANGE: INNER JOY

Prolific and abundant, orange blossom has the rare quality of bearing flowers and fruit simultaneously. To the ancient Chinese the translucent flowers symbolized youthfulness, sweetness and innocence, and they used the blossoms to adorn their brides' wedding regalia. The many seeds in the fruit suggest fruitfulness and fertility.

Orange blossom has been an ingredient in love potions throughout the ages and in many cultures. At the time of the Crusades, the Saracens gave it to brides to induce feelings of serenity and joy. In the eighteenth century English ladies drank "Angel Water" – an aphrodisiac punch containing orange blossom and rose water, which they believed made them irresistible to men.

Orange Blossom Essence Especially beneficial for mothers, this remedy banishes depression and relieves headaches. It renews hope, uplifts the spirit, brings joy and cultivates an "inner smile". In children it dispels sadness and discontentment, stops moodiness and brings out their sweet nature.

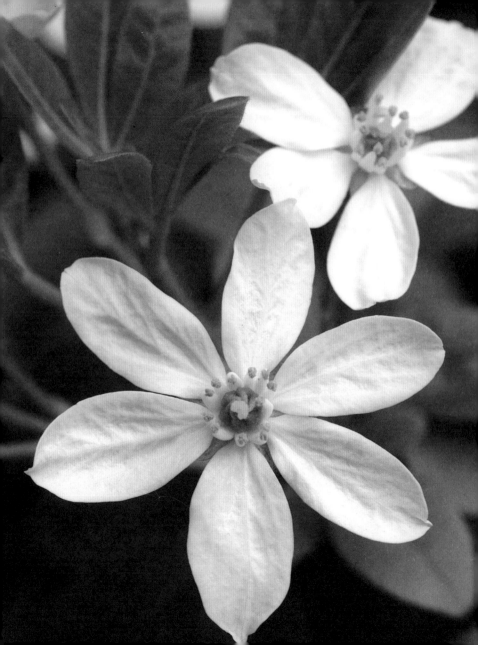

FRANGIPANI: THE JOY OF BEING A A WOMAN

The frangipani or plumera tree is a Buddhist symbol of immortality. Planted near temples, shrines and pagodas, it was known as the "the tree of life" because its flowers continue to bloom long after they have been cut from the mother plant. In Asia it is called the temple or pagoda tree and Hindus offer the flowers to the gods.

Highly respected and loved, frangipani is found in many sub-tropical and tropical regions. Growing throughout Polynesia, it is known as *pua melia* in Hawaii, where people love to weave the white and yellow, five-petalled flowers into floral garlands or *lei*s which they give in greeting. Frangipani has a sensuous fragrance and qualities of deep inner strength and beauty.

Frangipani Essence Celebrates the joy of being a woman and returns her to her original state of purity and innocence: the true "spirit of beauty".

Red Suva Frangipani Essence Restores inner calm after emotional turmoil and a relationship break-up.

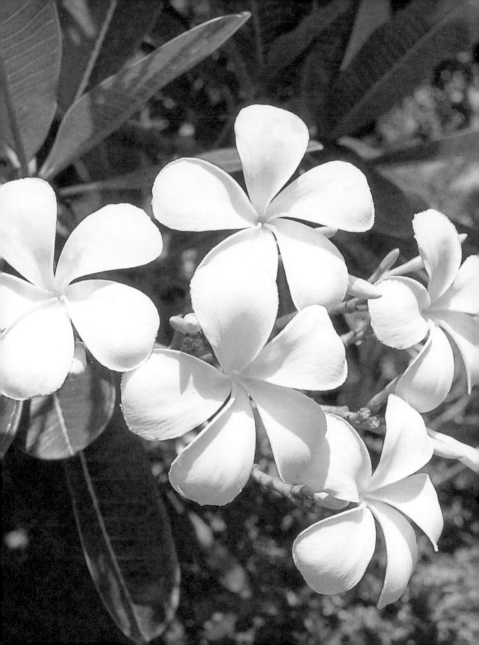

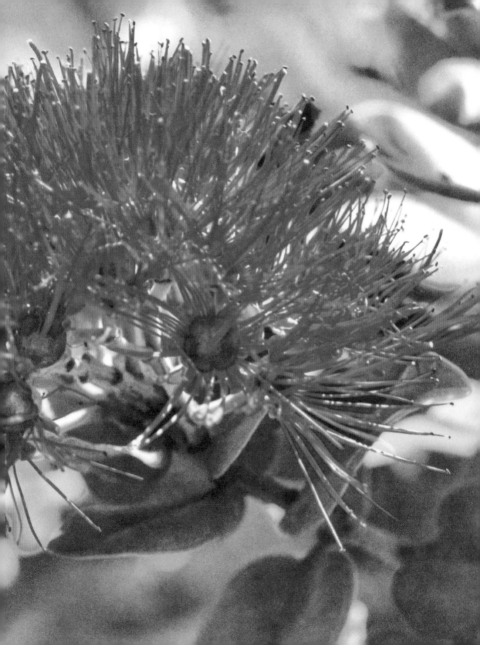

LEHUA: INNER PASSION

Lehua flowers bloom on *ohi'a* trees, which were the first trees to grow on the seven newly-formed islands of the fire goddess, Hawaii. The bright red, pom-pom flowers attracted the now rare, scarlet *i'iwi* bird, which loved their sweet fragrance and nectar. Lehua blooms are sacred to Pele, the fire goddess of the volcano. Pele's fiery, passionate spirit commanded great respect, as she embodies the positive life force and explosive energy rising from the core of the planet, symbolizing new birth and the abundant source of creativity.

Lovers wishing to ignite or rekindle the flames of passion would invoke her help by throwing offerings of vibrant lehua flowers into her volcano's fiery depths.

Hawaiian *huna* medicine men and women used lehua flowers to lessen the pain of childbirth.

Lehua Essence Its inner force and passion strengthens the female aspect, enhancing self-esteem by increasing sensuality. Restores, balances and liberates the female psyche by enhancing the activity of the sacral chakra.

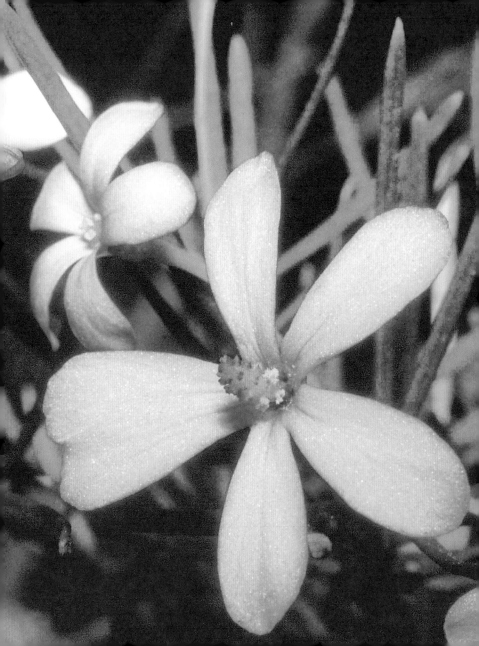

WEDDING BUSH: COMMITMENT

These beautiful, star-like flowers were used as romantic messengers by Aboriginal men and women in New South Wales. When a couple wished to marry they would exchange wedding bush flowers as an expression of their desire to wed. However, if they tired of each other, they had only to exchange the flowers for a second time and the marriage was over.

In the outback the early European settlers used the flowers to decorate brides' veils, and incorporated wedding bush flowers into their marriage ceremonies.

Wedding Bush Essence This is excellent for people who avoid responsibilities, and have difficulty in making a commitment, whether to a relationship or their own personal goals. It helps to form bonds, acting like invisible glue to hold a relationship together. It is also useful for people wishing to re-commit to each other, as well as for those wishing to break the cycle of jumping from one relationship to another. It supports our dedication to goals and grounds our life's purpose.

GARDENIA: COMMUNICATION

The gardenia, a symbol of sacred love and happiness, was used in weddings in Victorian times. This beautiful flower with its sensual fragrance was traditionally worn by daughters on Mother's Day. A red gardenia was worn if your mother was still alive, and a white gardenia if your mother had passed away.

Every morning the men of Tahiti pluck gardenias and wear them behind their ears. The flowers symbolize the "soul of Polynesia", where all that's good is free.

The bush gardenia of Australia is found in tropical woodlands in the Northern Territory.

Gardenia Essence This helps to deepen commitment in supportive relationships, increasing our awareness of the needs and desires of others. It initiates creativity and helps us to translate our ideas into reality.

Bush Gardenia Essence This is recommended to improve communications, and to renew interest and passion in male-female relationships where complacency and over-familiarity have set in.

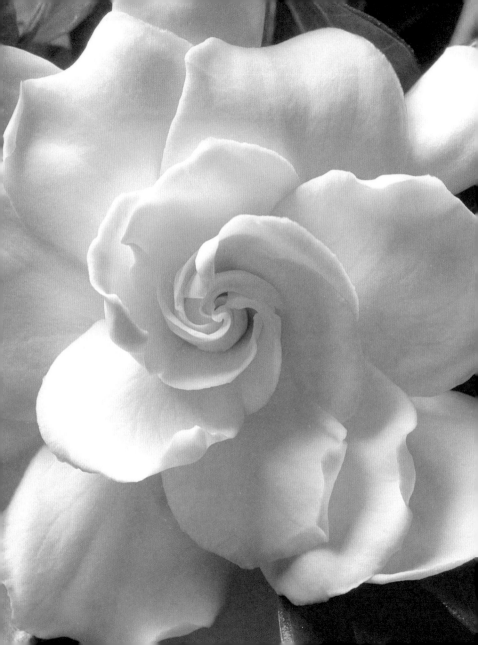

APPLE: A HEALTHY MINDSET

Apple trees and their fruits and flowers have enjoyed special significance in most cultures. The blossom is considered divine as its scented flowers are followed by crisp, thirst-quenching, life-giving fruit.

Mythology tells of the magical qualities of the golden apples of the Hesperides, which were found at the foot of Mount Atlas on the Island of the Blessed. The earth goddess Gaia presented them to Hera and Zeus as a wedding gift. According to Norse mythology, the goddess Idunn tended sacred apples, which were said to contain the secret of eternal youth – those deprived of their golden elixir aged rapidly.

In Egypt, the pharaoh Ramesses III offered 848 baskets of apples to Hapi, the fertility god of the Nile.

Apple Blossom Essence Promotes a healthy, positive attitude to life, clearing away worries, doubts and fears. In children, apple blossom remedy is very effective for treating emotional upsets and any kind of physical symptoms caused by stress.

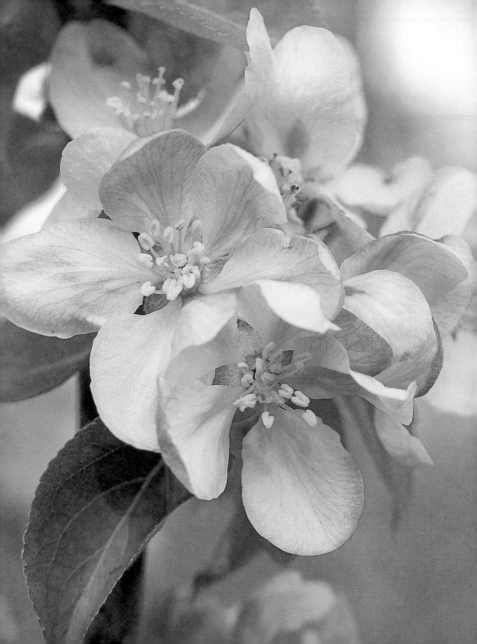

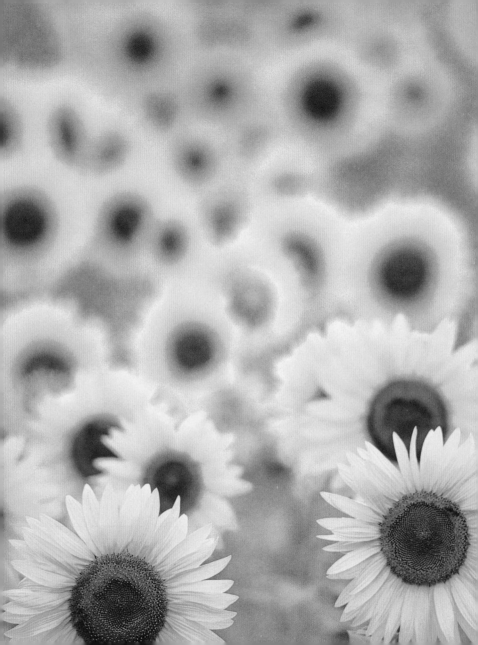

The goal of life is living in agreement with nature.

ZENO OF CITIUM

(C.335-263 BC)

The purpose of miracles is to teach us to see the
miraculous everywhere.

ST AUGUSTINE

(354-430 AD)

ROSE: LOVE AND ROMANCE

The rose graced the earth with its beautiful blooms thousands of years before the appearance of humankind. Evidence from fossils shows that it has existed since prehistoric times. Steeped in symbolism and myth, roses in the Garden of Eden are said to have blushed in shame when Adam and Eve were banished.

Originating in China, the romantic rose has symbolized the perfection of love and desire, both earthly and spiritual. The Egyptian queen Cleopatra is famed for her passion for bathing in milk and rose petals, and for filling her bed chamber with the petals when she had romantic rendezvous with Mark Anthony.

In ancient Greece, the flower goddess Cloris designated the rose "Queen of the Flowers." During festivals in Athens, young men and women crowned with garlands of roses danced naked near the temple of Hymen, symbolizing the innocence of the golden age. The red rose is the flower of Adonis, Eros and Cupid, while the white rose is sacred to Aphrodite and Venus.

To ancient magicians the seven-petalled rose signified degrees of absolute perfection, while the eight-petalled rose symbolized regeneration and rebirth.

Native peoples of the west coast of Canada would bury their loved ones with Nootka roses to guarantee them a protected, joyful passage into the next life. Native Americans saw the purity of the white rose as a sign of the happiness to come when they wore it during their wedding ceremonies.

Roses have always been messengers of love. In the language of flowers, a lavender rose – as a gift– denotes love at first sight; a coral rose implies desire; an orange rose conveys fascination and enthusiasm, and a pale pink rose means grace and admiration.

Rose perfume nourishes and enhances femininity, uplifting the heart, evoking sensual bliss and bringing spiritual purity.

Roses as a species are said to be highly evolved and they help us to return to the realms of the spirit.

Nootka Rose Essence Very effective for healing after trauma and dissolving bitterness. Particularly excellent after a spiritual crisis, it centres us in the heart, promoting laughter and happiness.

Tibetan Rock Rose Essence Helps us to love and appreciate ourselves as we are, reinforcing our zest for life.

Cherokee Rose Essence Balances the female endocrine system, allieviating women's problems.

Marie Pavie Rose Essence Encourages us to listen to our heart in relationships, and re-ignites passion.

Green Rose Essence Alleviates the negative effect of too much pressure and stress, and restores inner calm and detachment. It releases tension and widens our perception, helping us to develop, enhance and spiritualize our psychic abilities.

Old Blush Essence Increases our stamina, inner strength and calm. Enhances creative expression in all aspects of life.

Wild Rose Essence In a world full of obstacles, this rose encourages us to remain steadfast and true to our own convictions, helping us to reconnect with nature and develop a new zest for life. It restores our inner stability and power.

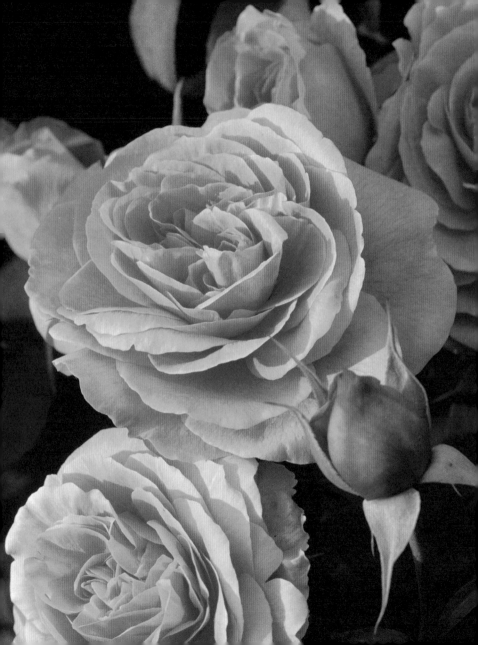

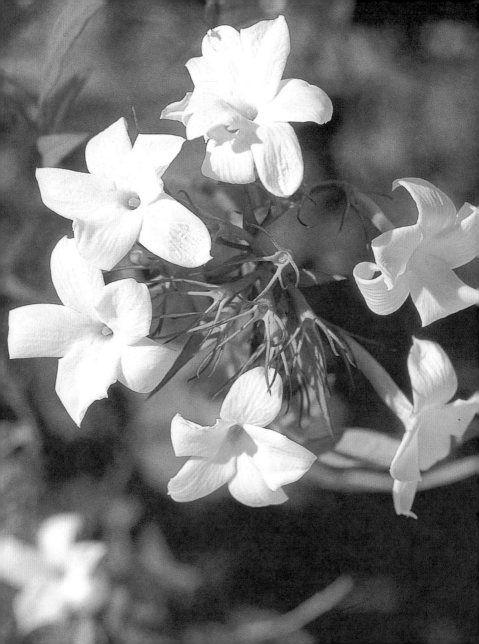

JASMINE: SENSUALITY

This delicate flower is associated with Isis, the ancient Egyptian goddess of fertility and compassionate mother goddess of the moon, who holds the secrets of healing and magic, and invented the custom of marriage.

Jasmine is a sacred plant in India. Kama, the Hindu god of love, who like Cupid is represented with a bow, was said to tip his arrows of desire with jasmine flowers. Known as "Queen of the Night" because its perfume intensifies after sunset, its voluptuous, warm fragrance is considered to be an aphrodisiac that awakens passion. Jasmine blossom is often woven into Indian brides' wedding garlands. Similarly, in south-east Asia, women interweave jasmine flowers into their newly washed and oiled hair to enhance sensuality.

Purple and White Jasmine Essence Harmonizes the sensual aspect of love with the emotional, helping to transmute physical love into spiritual love.

Night Jasmine Essence Attunes and synchronizes the sexual energies of couples before lovemaking.

WATERLILY: SENSUALITY, SEXUALITY AND SPIRITUALITY

The waterlily is a flower of love — beautiful to behold, with petals that are soft to touch and a sweet aroma that hangs in the warm air.

In the mythical land of Mu or Lemuria where life on earth is said to have begun, the waterlily was the first flower created and it became Mu's symbol. When the continent was submerged, the waterlily closed its petals in memory.

In ancient Buddhist tradition there were temples in Malaysia and Thailand specializing in flower essence healing and the waterlily was one of the major spiritual plants used. It was also an important flower in Balinese culture in which it symbolized wisdom and purity of heart. In Bali it was offered ceremonially to the gods.

Waterlilies are evocative of the sensuality and purity of love. These flowers come in a wonderful variety of species, from the stunningly beautiful, tropical magenta waterlilies that only open their petals in night air, to the delicate pink and white flowers found high up in the Himalayas. Perhaps the most magnificent species is the *Victoria Amazonica*, a gigantic waterlily found deep in the Amazon jungle.

In Central America the Mayan jaguar priests were represented by a jaguar playing with the waterlily as a symbol of divinity. Mayan shamans ingested the flower's juice to induce visions of becoming divine.

The ancient Egyptians also revered the waterlily. They marveled at the powerful vision of this pristine flower emerging in the morning from murky waters, only to sink again when the sun set. The blue waterlily was prized above all others and was considered to be the symbol of creation, as Ra, the Egyptian sun god, was said to have been born from its centre. The Egyptian high priests and royalty used the plant in a shamanic way to enhance perception and induce a positive state of unity.

In the Middle Ages the waterlily symbolized purity and virginity. If a love potion was employed to dissolve a maiden's resolve, she could remain chaste by carrying a waterlily in her hand.

Waterlily Essence Balances sensuality and sexuality with spirituality. Gently blends the energies of the heart and the sacral chakras. Allows a woman to be open to receive, yielding with softness and sensuality. Heightens sensations of touch, making her more aware of the softness of her own skin and body as well as encouraging the desire to express love through the sensuousness of touching.

Indian Waterlily Essence Eases fears of intimacy, heightens sensuality and enjoyment in love-making, and spiritualizes sexuality.

Night-blooming Waterlily Essence The essence of the shy, magenta, tropical flower that only opens its petals at night is ideal for enhancing love-making by creating a mystical atmosphere of love and romance.

Day-blooming Waterlily Essence The vibrant, purple, yellow-centred waterlily that only opens its petals during the day is perfect for harmonizing sexual energy by releasing any feelings of inadequacy, guilt or fear concerning sex. It encourages a positive attitude, enriching love-making, and emphasizes love and fulfilment.

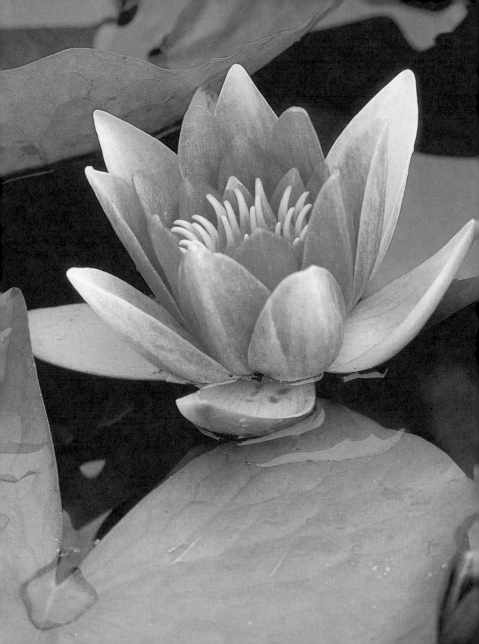

ORCHID: CONNECTION WITH SPIRIT

Orchids universally deliver the message of love, beauty and wisdom. The Far East is home to a stunning array of fine orchids. In China they signify enlightenment and child-like innocence and are dedicated to Quan Yin, the Chinese goddess of love and healing.

Orchids are one of the most exotic and prolific of the world's flowers. More than 25,000 different orchids have been catalogued, and new species are still being discovered. Orchids belong to the most recently evolved species of the plant kingdom. They have developed into a wonderful and fascinating variety of forms, with some adapting beyond the mere need for survival by visually mimicking the exact shape and scent of certain female insects and so attracting male insects to pollinate them.

In Europe orchids grow roots in the soil. However, those that grow in the Amazon and in the sub-tropical regions of Australia have developed roots that only take hold in the highest branches of the tree-tops in the rainforest canopy, where they can benefit from an optimum amount of light. To survive in the steamy rainforests, these large orchids growing high up on the bark of jungle trees need only support roots. They live independently of the trees they inhabit, and find nourishment through a symbiotic relationship with fungi.

The jungle shamans consider orchids to be the flowers closest to Spirit, perhaps because some of these spectacular blooms resemble angels and fairies, and also have the unique quality of seeming to live entirely on air. The ethereal properties of orchids are an indication of the use of these extraordinary flowers.

The shamans revere orchids as highly evolved flowers, believing they create a direct connection between human beings, the cosmos and the spiritual realms. They consider orchids to be able to accelerate humankind's spiritual evolution, connecting us to angels and spirits, and vibrating at a very high frequency that resonates with the subtle anatomy. They also acknowledge that the flowers harbour nature spirits which have a dynamic and otherworldly effect on sexual energy, heightening awareness of the divine aspect of sexuality.

Orchid Queen Essence Designed specially to enable women to tap into free-flowing, magnetic energy, it heals the female psyche, inspiring wonder at being a woman, and touching the heart and mind with joy.

Heart Orchid Essence Strengthens and harmonizes the heart and solar plexus chakras by transmuting negative, self-centred emotions into positive energy through the power of love.

Angel of Protection Orchid Essence Enhances communication with our guardian angels and acts a protective shield for sensitive people exposed to hostile environments.

Sun Orchid Cream A beauty cream for dry, sensitive skin created with Sun Orchid and Angel Orchid essences to uplift, lighten and express a woman's inner beauty.

Dancing Orchid Cream A beauty cream for sensitive combination skin, with Orchid Queen and Lotus essences to nurture a woman's self-confidence and feeling of grace and beauty. It is blended with rose and jasmine oils to clear and balance the skin, helping to achieve a soft, dewy complexion.

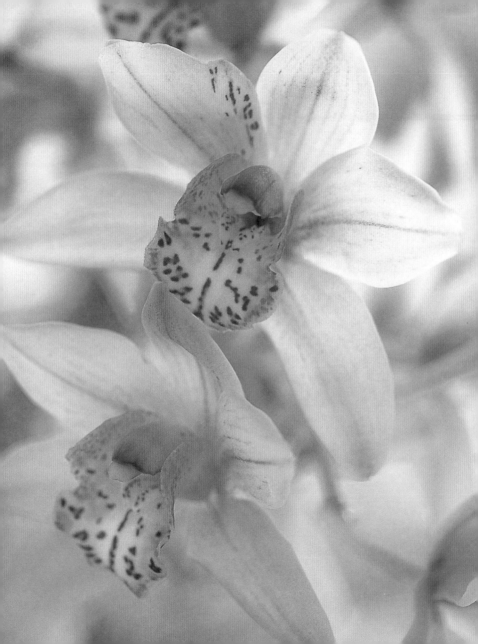

This is the spirit that is in my heart, smaller than a
grain of rice ... or a grain of canary-seed, or the kernel
of a grain of canary-seed; this is the spirit that is in my
heart, greater than the Earth ... greater than heaven
itself, greater than all these worlds.

UPANISHADS

(C.1000 BC)

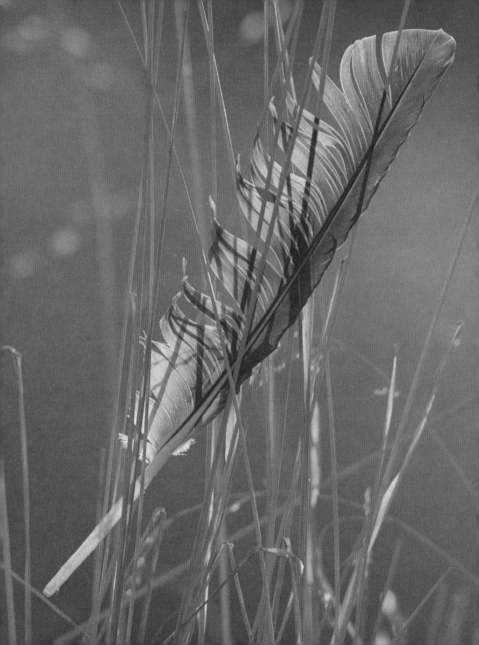

LILY: SIMPLICITY AND INTEGRATION

In ancient Greece and Rome a garland of white lilies – a symbol of purity, fertility and abundance – was placed on the bride's head during wedding ceremonies.This lily was associated with Juno, Jupiter and Venus. According to legend, Venus saw a beautiful white lily as she rose from the sea and because she felt it rivalled her own beauty, she created a large yellow pistil in its snow white centre.

In China the lily was an emblem of motherhood and to dream of these flowers in the springtime denoted a happy marriage.

Early representations of the lily were discovered in Crete. It was sacred flower of the ancient Minoans and was associated with Britomartis, their goddess of hunting and the moon.

A Christian legend tells of the first lily springing from the tears of Eve as she sadly left the Garden of Eden. The white lily was originally used by artists to illustrate the heavenly delights and marvels of paradise.

Later, it came to be associated with the Madonna, symbolizing the mystery of the virgin birth. The Madonna lily is loved for its majestic air and heady scent. It also became an emblem of the saints because of its ability to help develop purity and humility.

The Lily encourages not only purity but the nurturing and feminine qualities of peace and calm as well as bringing the sacred feminine into the soul of both men and women.

There are a huge variety of lilies from the spectacular giant lily to the delicate lily of the valley. The humble lily of the valley has a gentle, calming fragrance and is associated with Ostara, the Norse goddess of springtime. English folklore tells of the origins of the lily of the valley in the legend of Saint Leonard and Sin, a dragon. Representing good and evil respectively, they fought for three days. On the fourth day good triumphed and Sin crept off into the forest to lick his wounds. However, Saint Leonard, too, was grievously injured and wherever droplets of his blood fell, lilies of the valley sprang up as a symbols of his goodness and purity.

Paradise Lily Remedy Reawakens our connection to the higher realms. Aids meditation, strengthens our inner awareness and consciousness of the divine.

Mariposa Lily Remedy Enhances maternal feelings and mother-child bonding. Heals the inner child and anyone with feelings of childhood abandonment or abuse.

Calla Lily Remedy Restores balance helping to integrate our masculine (active) and feminine (receptive) aspects. Enhances self worth and creativity.

Fire Lily Remedy Promotes a healthy and loving attitude towards intimacy when appropriate. Activates the creative forces, giving us the ability to overcome any obstacles that prevent fulfillment of our goals.

Lily of the Valley Remedy Helps us to see through the eyes of a child, returning us to the innocent state where responding with simplicity from a place of trust is the only loving response possible.

Easter Lily Remedy Integrates different aspects of the personality, encouraging honesty and openness. Works on the kidney energy in Chinese medicine and has proved effective for treating PMT in women.

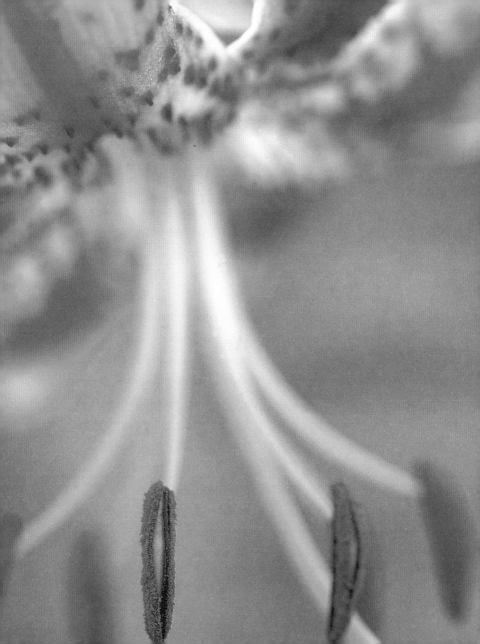

LOTUS: ENLIGHTENMENT

The lotus is considered to be the most spiritual and sacred of all flowers in most of the countries of the Far East and in Australia. A flower of such purity and perfection that it is said to hold the wisdom of the world, the lotus was given its name when Neptune's beautiful daughter Lotis was transformed into a lotus plant by the gods, when they were seeking to keep her safe from the lustful eyes of Priapus, a personification of male sexual power.

The ancient Egyptian legend of the white lotus describes it as the first flower to appear on the earth. In Egypt it became a symbol of new life, decorating the altars of the gods. According to records the pharaoh Ramesses III presented as many as 3,410 lotus garlands to the gods in the temple of Amun as his personal offering. The leaves and flowers of the lotus plant were said to have euphoric qualities when ingested, and it was believed to encourage the dying to seek the highest possible reincarnation their next life.

In Hindu mythology it is said that before creation the world was a golden lotus: the Madripadma or Mother Lotus. This Mother Lotus is considered to be the mystical birth place of Lord Brahma and it symbolizes his magical powers. In India it is depicted growing from the navel of Lord Vishnu and heralds the birth of the universe born from a central sun.

The flower was also so significant to Buddhists that they named it the Thousand-petalled Lotus, and the Buddha is often shown sitting in the calyx of the flower.

The qualities of the lotus were well recognized and appreciated by the Aborigines in Australia, where a large lotus with deep pink fragrant flowers and a yellow centre grows in the billabongs of the flood plains.

The lotus was chosen to symbolize spiritual enlightenment, because the vision of this perfect and exquisite flower rising out of mud and murky waters gives humankind hope that, out of chaos, something pure, wonderful and eminently spiritual can grow.

The qualities emanating from this spiritual flower are so powerful that it is considered sacred wherever it grows and is perceived to possess wisdom that goes beyond time itself – even its seeds are long-lived with some germinating only after 200 years.

Lotus Essence As the flower of enlightenment and wisdom, the lotus produces a profoundly powerful essence, promoting clarity and enlightenment. Lotus essence treats all aspects of a person, harmonizing and balancing all the chakras, meridians and the subtle anatomy. In realigning the entire system, it initiates positive energy changes, ridding the body of unhealthy patterns of illness, emotional and physical toxins by gently bringing them to the surface to be cleared.

Lotus corrects emotional imbalances, calms the mind, and improves concentration and focus. It is excellent for meditation and creative visualization because it stimulates, harmonizes and redirect the energy of the crown chakra, the gateway to higher consciousness. This integrates the whole being. Lotus essence accelerate humankind's spiritual evolvement and deepens our insight and understanding of the purpose of our souls the earthly plane.

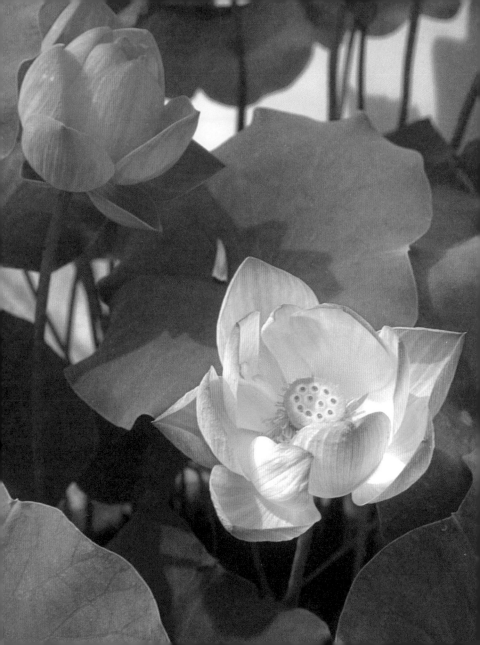

BUYING AND STORING ESSENCES

Flower essences are readily available from most good health-food stores and you can also buy them through mail order and online (see p.125).

When storing essences it is best to keep them away from strong light and products such as homeopathic remedies, herbal medicines and essential oils. The usual dosage is seven drops taken just before you go to sleep and as soon as you wake up, so it is a good idea to keep your dropper bottles by your bed to make it easy to remember to take your essences. Again, keep them away from oils, medicines and perfumes. It is not advisable to keep essences in the bathroom or in your make-up bag (except Emergency Essence in your handbag or pocket) as strong substances can affect their energetic qualities.

Flower essences are easy to use, and if you need to take them more often than first thing in the morning and last thing at night, you do not need to take into consideration whether you have or have not eaten or drunk anything, as they are effective taken at any time.

CONCLUSION

There is no doubt that flowers have held a special place in our hearts since the beginning of time. But they also have the power to make a major impact by stimulating radical changes in our lives.

Since working professionally with flower remedies over the last twenty years, I have had the privilege of witnessing the extraordinary and profound changes – whether physical, emotional, mental or spiritual – that the essences have helped to initiate in my clients. For some people changing takes great courage, faith and energy to enable the process of re-establishing wellness and balance to begin, especially when they have faced dramatic or life-threatening challenges.

I never cease to marvel at the versatility and sheer tenacity of spirit in flower essences, and their gentle yet profoundly supportive effect on us.

Life would be a soulless place without these beautiful expressions of nature. Their healing essence is nature's gift to humankind.

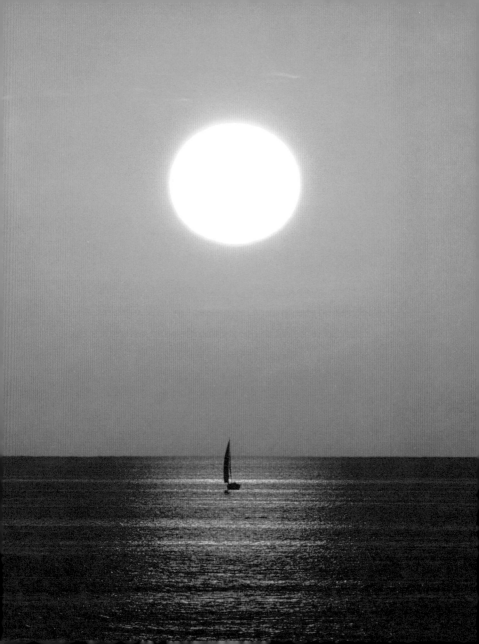

The wind of God's grace is incessantly blowing. Lazy
sailors on the sea of life do not take advantage of it. But
the active and the strong always keep the sails of their
minds unfurled to catch the favourable wind and thus
reach their destination very soon.

SRI RAMAKRISHNA

(1836-88)

FLOWER ESSENCE PRODUCERS

The Producers

Aum Himalaya
  Essences **[AumH]**
Australian Bush
  Essences **[AusB]**
Australian Living
  Essences **[AusL]**
Spirit of Beauty /
  Clare G Harvey's
  Skincare Range **[SPB]**
Flower Essence
  Services **[FES]**
Flowers of the Orient
  [FO]
Gaia Hawiian **[Haii]**
Korte PHI **[AK]**
Master's Essences **[MA]**
Pacific Essences **[Pac]**
Petite Fleur Essences
  [PF]

Single Flower Essences

Sage **[AK]**
Aloe Vera **[FES, AK]**
Hibiscus **[FO]**
Red Hibiscus **[AK]**
Sturt Desert Pea **[AusB]**
Waratah **[AusB]**
Self-heal **[FES]**
Almond Blossom **[MA]**
Magnolia **[Pac]**
Japanese Magnolia **[PF]**
Bird of Paradise **[AK]**
Iris **[FES]**
Daisy **[AK]**
Boab **[AusB]**

Cherry Blossom **[MA]**
Orange Blossom **[MA]**
Wild Violet **[AusL]**
Frangipani **[FO]**
Red Suva Frangipani
  [AusB]
Lehua **[Haii]**
Wedding Bush **[AusB]**
Gardenia **[PF]**
Bush Gardenia **[AusB]**
Apple Blossom **[MA]**
Nootka Rose **[Pac]**
Tibetan Rock Rose **[AK]**
Cherokee Rose **[PF]**
Marie Pervi Rose **[PF]**
Green Rose **[AK]**
Old Blush Rose **[PF]**
Wild Rose **[AK]**
Purple and White Jasmine
  [AumH]
Night Jasmine **[AumH]**
Waterlily **[FO]**
Indian Waterlily **[AumH]**
  Night / Day Blooming
  Waterlily **[AumH]**
Orchid Queen **[FO]**
Heart Orchid **[AK]**
Angel of Protection
  Orchid **[AK]**
Paradise Lily **[AK]**
Mariposa Lily **[Pac]**
Calla Lily **[AK]**
Fire Lily **[AK]**
Lily of the Valley **[Pac]**
Easter Lily **[Pac]**
Lotus **[AumH & AK]**

Combinations

Emergency Essence
  [AusB]
Dynamis Essence
  [AusB]
Cognis Essence **[AusB]**
Woman Essence **[AusB]**
Calm and Clear Essence
  [AusB]
Electro Essence **[AusB]**
Travel Essence **[AusB]**
Stop Smoking Blend **[PF]**
Reduce Stress Blend **[PF]**
Allergy / Intolerance
  Blend **[PF]**

Spritzes

Space Clearing Spray
  [AusB]
Spirit Lift Spray **[FO]**
Harmony and Balance
  Spray **[PF]**

Creams

Bird of Paradise Cream
  [SPB]
Self-heal Cream **[FES]**
Dancing Orchid Cream
  [SPB]
Sun Orchid Cream **[SPB]**
Floral Relief Gel
  [AumH]
Floral Arthritis Gel
  [AumH]

FLOWER ESSENCE SUPPLIERS

UK

Flowersense
19 London End
Beaconsfield
Bucks, HP9 2HN
tel: (01494) 671775 / (020) 8567 9412 /
(01963) 250750
email: info@flowersense.co.uk
www.flowersense.co.uk

Lines available: Aum Himalaya,
Australian Bush, Australian Living,
Spirit of Beauty / Clare G Harvey's
Skincare Range, FES, Flowers of the
Orient, Korte PHI, Master's, Petite Fleur.

Gaia Hawaiian Essences
28 Glebe Lands Road
Tiverton
Devon, EX16 4EB
tel: (01884) 259130
www.gaiaessences.com

USA

Flower Essence Services
PO Box 459
Nevada City
CA 95959,
tel: (530) 265 9163
www.fesflowers.com

Master's Essences
14618 Tyler Foote Rd
Nevada City
CA 95959,
tel: (530) 478 7655
www.mastersessences.com

Petite Fleur Essences
8524 Whispering Creek Trail
Fort Worth
Texas 76134
tel: (817) 293 5410
www.aromahealthtexus.com

CANADA

Pacific Essences
PO Box 8317
Victoria BC V8W3R9
tel: (250) 384 5560
www.pacificessences.com

AUSTRALIA

Australian Bush Essences
45 Booralie Rd
Terry Hills, NSW 2084
tel: (02) 9450 1388
www.ausflowers.com.au

INDIA

Aum Himalaya Essences
15E Jaybharat Society
3rd Road, Khar (West)
Mumbai 400052
tel: (22) 26486819
www.aumhimalaya.com

NETHERLANDS

Korte PHI Esences
Rijksweg Zuid 1
AM Belfeld, NL 5951
tel: (77) 475 4252
www.phiessences.com

INDEX

Contact the Author

Clare G. Harvey can be contacted by email at clare@flowersense.co.uk. For consultations with Clare in her London clinic in Upper Harley Street, W1, please phone (020) 7935 7848.

For information on Diploma Courses in Flower Essences, please phone (01963) 250750 or email info@vibrationalmedicine.co.uk.

Picture Credits

The publisher would like to thank the following people and photographic libraries for permission to reproduce their material. Every care has been taken to trace copyright holders. However, if we have omitted anyone we apologize and will, if informed, make corrections in any future edition.

Page 1 Torie Chugg/Andrew Lawson Photography; **2** Torie Chugg/Andrew Lawson Photography; **3** Richard Katz/Flower Essence Society; **19** Adam Jones/Image Bank/Getty Images; **21** Erich Lessing/AKG; **24** Penny Tweedie/Corbis; **30** Dinesh Khanna/Axiom; **35** Neovision/Getty Images; **43** Photodisc Collection/Getty Images; **46** Richard Katz/Flower Essence Society; **49** Cathie Welchman/Gaia Essences; **51** Andrew Lawson Photography; **54** Michael & Patricia Fogden/Corbis; **59** Clay Perry/Corbis; **61** Marianne Majerus Photography; **62** Ann Cutting/Photonica/Getty Images; **64** Marianne Majerus Photography ; **67** Harpur Garden Library; **69** Andrew Lawson Photography; **71** Mark Bolton/Corbis; **73** Torie Chugg/Andrew Lawson Photography; **74** Australian Bush Essences; **77** Andrew Lawson Photography; **79** Andrew Lawson Photography; **81** Marianne Majerus Photography; **83** Mark Bolton/Corbis; **85** Andrew Lawson Photography; **86** Cathie Welchman/ Gaia Essences; **88** Australian Bush Essences; **91** Clay Perry/Corbis; **93** Andrew Lawson Photography; **94** Jeremy Walker/Photographer's Choice/Getty Images; **99** Marianne Majerus Photography; **100** Harpur Garden Library; **105** Harpur Garden Library; **109** Torie Chugg/Andrew Lawson Photography; **111** Photolink/Getty Images; **115** Torie Chugg/ Andrew Lawson Photography; **119** Dave G. Houser/Post Houserstock/Corbis; **122** Frank Cezus/Photographer's Choice/Getty Images

Author's Acknowledgments

A big thank you to Grace Cheetham for her inspiration, and to Ingrid, Justin and all at Duncan Baird for creating a stunning book to be proud of.

Blessings to my mother Eliana Harvey, who added her insight and wisdom when I was writing this book.

Special thanks to Ian White, Andreas Korte, Lila Devi Stone, Judy Griffin, Richard Katz and Patricia Kaminski, Sabina Pettitt, Vasudeva and Kadambii Barnao, Rupa and Atul Shah, Cathie Welchman and all the rest of the flower essence family for their dedication and pioneering.